Unit Operations in
Pharmaceutical
Engineering

W0081068

Unit Operations in Pharmaceutical Engineering

Yasmin Sultana MPharm, PhD
Associate Professor
Department of Pharmaceutics
School of Pharmaceutical Education and Research
Jamia Hamdard
New Delhi

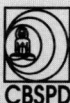

CBSPD

CBS Publishers & Distributors Pvt Ltd

New Delhi • Bengaluru • Chennai • Kochi • Kolkata • Lucknow • Mumbai
Hyderabad • Jharkhand • Nagpur • Patna • Pune • Uttarakhand

Disclaimer

Science and technology are constantly changing fields. New research and experience broaden the scope of information and knowledge. The author has tried her best in giving information available to her while preparing the material for this book. Although all efforts have been made to ensure optimum accuracy of the material, yet it is quite possible some errors might have been left uncorrected. The publisher, the printer and the author will not be held responsible for any inadvertent errors or inaccuracies.

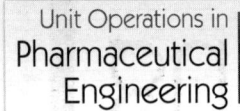

ISBN: 978-93-88178-95-2

Copyright © Author and Publisher

First Edition: 2019
Reprint: 2022, 2024

All rights reserved. No part of this book may be reproduced or transmitted in any form or by any means, electronic or mechanical, including photocopying, recording, or any information storage and retrieval system without permission, in writing, from the author and the publisher.

Published by **Satish Kumar Jain** and produced by **Varun Jain** for

CBS Publishers & Distributors Pvt Ltd

4819/XI Prahlad Street, 24 Ansari Road, Daryaganj, New Delhi 110 002, India.

Ph: 011-23289259, 23266861

Website: www.cbspd.com
e-mail: delhi@cbspd.com

Corporate Office: 204 FIE, Industrial Area, Patparganj, Delhi 110 092

Ph: 011-4934 4934   Fax: 011-4934 4935 e-mail: publishing@cbspd.com;publicity@cbspd.com

Branches

- Bengaluru: Seema House 2975, 17th Cross, K.R. Road, Banasankari 2nd Stage, Bengaluru 560 070 Karnataka, India
  Ph: +91-80-26771678/79   Fax: +91-80-26771680   e-mail: bangalore@cbspd.com
- Chennai: 7, Subbaraya Street, Shenoy Nagar, Chennai 600 030, Tamil Nadu, India
  Ph: +91-44-26680620, 26681266   Fax: +91-44-42032115   e-mail: chennai@cbspd.com
- Kochi: 42/1325, 1326, Power House Road, Opp KSEB, Ernakulam 682 018, Kochi, Kerala, India
  Ph: +91-484-4059061-67   Fax: +91-484-4059065   e-mail: kochi@cbspd.com
- Kolkata: 147, Hind Ceramics Compound, 1st Floor, Nilgunj Road, Belghoria, Kolkata 700 056, West Bengal, India
  Ph: + 91-33-25633055/56   e-mail: kolkata@cbspd.com
- Lucknow: Basement, Khushnuma Complex, 7-Meerabai Marg (Behind Jawahar Bhawan), Lucknow 226 001, UP, India
  Ph: + 0552-4000032   e-mail: tiwari.lucknowi@cbspd.com
- Mumbai: PWD Shed. Gala no. 25/26, Ramchandra Bhatt Marg, Next to JJ Hospital Gate no. 2, Opp. Union Bank of India, Noorbaug, Mumbai 400 009, Maharashtra, India
  Ph: 022-66661880/89   e-mail: mumbai@cbspd.com

Representatives

• Hyderabad	0-9885175004	• Jharkhand	0-9811541605	• **Nagpur**	0-8692091830
• Patna	0-9334159340	• Pune	0-9664372571	• **Uttarakhand**	0-9716462459

Printed at Rashtriya Printers, Dilshad Garden, Delhi, India

Contributors

Atefeh Afshar Moghaddam M Pharm, PhD
Research Scholar
Department of Pharmaceutics
SPER, Jamia Hamdard
New Delhi, India

Iram Aliya Khan M Pharm
Research Scholar
Department of Pharmaceutics
SPER, Jamia Hamdard
New Delhi, India

Jayamanti Pandit M Pharm, PhD
Assistant Professor
Department of Pharmaceutics
K.R. Mangalam University, Gurgaon, India

Mahfooz Rahman M Pharm, PhD
Assistant Professor
Department of Pharmaceutical Sciences
Faculty of Health Sciences
SHUATS, Allahabad, India

Manju Sharma M Pharm, PhD
Associate Professor
Department of Pharmacology
SPER, Jamia Hamdard
New Delhi, India

Md Shakeeb Ahmed M Pharm
Research Scholar
Department of Pharmaceutics
SPER, Jamia Hamdard
New Delhi, India

Meenakshi Chauhan M Pharm, PhD
Associate Professor
Department of Pharmaceutics, DIPSARU
New Delhi, India

Md AbulKalam M Pharm, PhD
Assistant Professor
Department of Pharmaceutics
College of Pharmacy
King Saud University
Riyadh, Saudi Arabia

Md Aqil M Pharm, PhD
Associate Professor
Department of Pharmaceutics
SPER, Jamia Hamdard
New Delhi, India

Nikita M Pharm
Research Scholar
Department of Pharmaceutics
SPER, Jamia Hamdard
New Delhi, India

Saima Amin M Pharm, PhD
Assistant Professor
Department of Pharmaceutics
SPER, Jamia Hamdard
New Delhi, India

Syed Mahmood M Pharm, PhD
Senior lecturer
Department of Manufacturing
(Pharmaceutical Engineering)
Faculty of Engineering Technology
University Malaysia Pahang
Kuantan, Pahang
Malaysia

Thasleem M M Pharm
Research Scholar
Department of Pharmaceutics
SPER, Jamia Hamdard
New Delhi, India

Preface

*U*nit *Operations in Pharmaceutical Engineering* is a textbook meant for B Pharm Semester III students, based on the revised syllabus laid down by Pharmacy Council of India. The primary objective of this book is to present the basic principles of unit operations in an easy and effective manner. The evolution of this book is a result of my years of teaching this subject to the undergraduate students of pharmacy. The material presented in this book is simplified to give the reader a clear and complete understanding of the subject. Although efforts are made to design the contents strictly as per syllabus, but for promotion of better understanding certain details are included to make it more interesting.

I acknowledge with gratitude the helpful comments and suggestions from colleagues, fellow teachers and students. I would like to thank Iram, Nikita, Shakeeb, Pavitra and Pramod for their help in proofreading. While every effort has been made to minimize errors, some errors may have been overlooked. Your feedback will be highly appreciated.

Yasmin Sultana

Contents

Flow of Fluids

Meenakshi Chauhan and Yasmin Sultana

FLUID MECHANICS

Fluid mechanics is the study of fluids and the forces on them. Fluids include liquids, gases, and plasmas. Fluid mechanics is classified into: fluid kinematics, the study of fluid motion, and fluid dynamics, the study of the effect of forces on fluid motion, which can further be divided into fluid statics, the study of fluids at rest, and fluid kinetics, the study of fluids in motion (Fig. 1.1). It is a branch of continuum mechanics which is a subject that models matter without using the information that it is been made out of atoms. Its models does not matter from a microscopic view point but rather than matter from a macroscopic viewpoint.

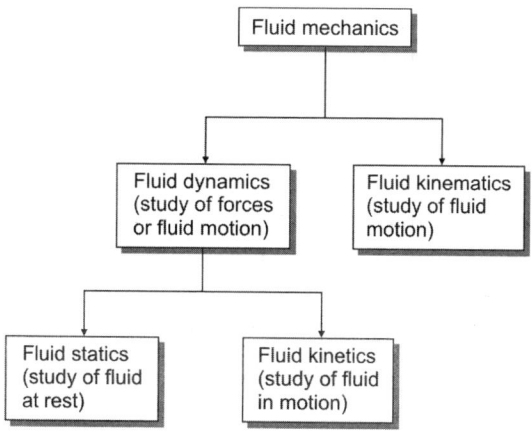

Fig. 1.1: Fluid mechanics (scheme)

A fluid is a substance which can flow. A continuous relative motion between different particles of a substance is the description of flow in technical terms. Under influence of shear forces the relative motion between particles make the fluid to flow. The particles starts moving when they cannot resist the shear force. Under shear stress a fluid without returning to its original position can deform indefinitely.

A fluid is defined as a material continuum which is unable to withstand a static shear stress. A fluid responds with an irrecoverable flow unlike an elastic solid which responds to a shear stress with a recoverable deformation. Variables needed to define a fluid and its environment are shown in Table 1.1

Table 1.1: Variables needed to define a fluid and its environment

Quantity	Symbol	Object	Units
Pressure	P	Scalar	N/m^2
Velocity	V	Vector	m/s
Density	R	Scalar	kg/m^3
Viscosity	M	Scalar	kg/m-s
Body force	B	Vector	N/kg
Time	T	Scalar	S

Euler Equations
In fluid dynamics, the Euler equations govern the motion of a compressible, inviscid fluid. They correspond to the Navier-Stokes equations with zero viscosity. They directly represent conservation of mass, momentum, and energy.

Laplace's Equation
The Laplace equations describes the behaviour of gravitational, electric, and fluid potentials.

The Bernoulli Equation
A statement of the conservation of energy in a form useful for solving problems involving fluids. For a non-viscous, incompressible fluid in steady flow, the sum of pressure, potential and kinetic energies per unit volume is constant at any point.

Conservation Laws
- The conservation laws states that particular measurable properties of an isolated physical system do not change as the system evolves.
- Conservation of energy (including mass)
- Fluid mechanics and conservation of mass—The law of conservation of mass states that mass can neither be created nor destroyed.
- The continuity equation—It is a statement that mass is conserved.

Ideal Gas Law
- The ideal gas law—For a perfect or ideal gas the change in density is directly related to the change in temperature and pressure as expressed in the ideal gas law.
- Properties of gas mixtures—Special care must be taken for gas mixtures when using the ideal gas law, calculating the mass, the individual gas constant or the density.
- The individual and universal gas constant—It is common in fluid mechanics and thermodynamics.

Navier-Stokes Equations

The motion of a non-turbulent, Newtonian fluid is governed by the Navier-Stokes equations. The equation can be used to model turbulent flow, where the fluid parameters are interpreted as time-averaged values.

PROPERTIES OF FLUIDS

The term fluid includes both liquid and gases. Whereas, liquids are considered to be incompressible, while gases are considered to be compressible.

A liquid can takes the shape of a surface in contact and a gas completely occupies the available space. As the liquid is the fluid for consideration in hydraulics so we examine properties of the liquid.

Mass density: It is the mass of the fluid per unit volume. Its unit is kg per cubic meter.

Specific weight: It is the weight per unit volume of fluid. Its units are Newton per cubic meter.

Compressibility: The property of the fluid by virtue of which its volume decrease on application of pressure is called compressibility.

Elasticity: The property by virtue of it the fluid returns to its original volume, when the force which is generating pressure is released.

Vapour pressure: Vapour pressure of the liquid is the pressure which is attained when molecule of liquid escape from surface to fill the space above the liquid surface and container till their pressure is equal to pressures due to these molecules.

Surface tension: Surface tension is caused due to cohesive force between molecules of the liquid, it is the weak force at the interface between liquid and air.

Capillarity: There are two type of forces acting on molecules of liquid. Cohesive forces are forces acting on molecules of liquid and adhesive forces are forces acting between liquid and container walls. When adhesive forces are greater than cohesive forces, liquid sticks to the wall of the container and results in capillary rise. When cohesion is more than adhesion, the capillary level dips.

Types of Fluids—Newtonian and Non-Newtonian Fluids

Those fluids which shows linear relationship between shearing stress and rate of shearing strain. Shear actions, such as agitation or pumping at a constant temperature do not change viscosity r consistency of Newtonian liquids, hence they are called true liquids. Some example of Newtonian fluids are water and oils.

A Newtonian fluid the term coined by Isaac Newton which is defined to be a fluid whose shear stress is linearly proportional to the velocity gradient in the direction perpendicular to the plane of shear. This definition means no matter of the forces acting on a fluid as it *continues to flow*. For example, water is a Newtonian fluid as it continues to display its fluid properties regardless of how much it is stirred or mixed. Under normal conditions important fluids and most gases behaves as a Newtonian fluid.

Non Newtonian fluids are exemplified by materials, such as pudding, which while stirring leaves a hole which gradually fills up overtime.

Equations for a Newtonian Fluid

The proportionality constant between the shear stress and the velocity gradient is known as the viscosity. A simplest equation to describe Newtonian fluid behaviour is:

$$\tau = \mu v$$

where,

τ = shear stress exerted by the fluid ("drag")

μ = fluid viscosity (a constant of proportionality)

v = velocity gradient perpendicular to the direction of shear.

The viscosity of a Newtonian fluid does not depend on forces acting upon it, and depends on temperature and pressure.

Fluids are of two types: Ideal and non-ideal fluids. An ideal fluid does not exists in reality but in some calculations this assumption is justified. An ideal fluid is not viscous and offer no resistance to shearing force. Real fluids are of two types, Newtonian and non-Newtonian. Newtonian fluids agree with Newton's Law of viscosity while non-Newtonian liquids can be plastic, pseudoplastic, dilatant, thixotropic and rheopectic and viscoelastic.

Shear-thinning/pseudoplastic liquids: Shear-thinning or pseudoplastic liquids are those whose apparent viscosity decreases with increasing shear rate. Their structure is time-independent.

Thixotropic fluids: Thixotropic liquids have a time-dependent structure. The apparent viscosity of a thixotropic liquid decreases with increasing time, at a constant shear rate.

Example: Ketchup and mayonnaise are thixotropic materials that appear thick or viscous but are quite easily possible to pump.

Dilatant fluids: These are also known as shear thickening fluids which increase their viscosity with agitation. Some of these liquids can even become almost solid within a pump or pipe line. Cream becomes butter with agitation and even candy compounds, clay slurries and similar heavily filled liquids do bexhibit same behaviour.

Bingham plastic fluids: They have a yield value which must be exceeded before it will start to flow like a fluid. And from that point the viscosity will decrease with increase in agitation, e.g. toothpaste, mayonnaise and tomato ketchup.

Basic Equations of Fluid Flow

Viscosity: It is a measure of resistance to the flow of fluids and it defines the interaction between moving particles of the fluid. Due to difference in viscosity, the flow or rate of deformation of fluids under shear stress is different for different fluids.

The viscosity of a fluid is an essential property in the analysis of liquid behaviour and in fluid motion near solid boundaries. The fluid resistance is viscosity that is to shear or flow and is used to measure the adhesive/cohesive or frictional fluid property. The intermolecular friction causes resistance which is exerted when layers of fluids attempt to slide by one another. For proper design of required temperatures for storage, pumping or injection of fluids, the knowledge of viscosity is needed.

The fluid viscosity can be measured by dynamic (or absolute) and kinematic viscosity. Absolute or dynamic viscosity is the tangential force per unit area which is required to move one horizontal plane with respect to the other at unit velocity while maintaining a unit distance apart by the fluid (Fig. 1.2). The dynamic or absolute viscosity can be expressed as:

$$\tau = \mu \, dc/dy$$

Equation is known as the **Newtons Law of Friction**.

where,

τ = shearing stress

μ = dynamic viscosity

In the SI system the dynamic viscosity units are **N s/m²**, **Pa s** or **kg/m s**, where 1 *Pa s* = 1 N s/m² = 1 kg/m s

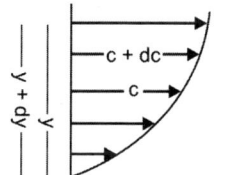

Fig. 1.2: Dynamic viscosity

The dynamic viscosity is often expressed in the metric CGS (centimeter-gram-second) system as *g/cm.s*, *dyne.s/cm²* or *poise (p)*, where 1 *poise* = *dyne s/cm²* = *g/cm s* = 1/10 *Pa s*

To use practically, the *Poise* is too large and its usually divided by *100* into the smaller unit called the *centi Poise (cP)*, where 1 *p* = 100 *cP*.

For example: Water at 68.4°F (20.2°C) has an absolute viscosity of one -1-*centi-poise*.

Kinematic Viscosity: It is defined as a ratio of absolute or dynamic viscosity to density, i.e. a quantity in which no force is involved. Kinematic viscosity can be obtained by dividing the absolute viscosity of a fluid by its mass density.

$$v = \mu/\rho$$

where,

v = kinematic viscosity

μ = absolute or dynamic viscosity

ρ = density

In the SI-system the theoretical unit is m²/s or commonly used *Stoke (St) Where,* 1 *St* = 10^{-4} m²/s.

Since, the *Stoke* is an impractical large unit, it is usual divided by *100* to give the unit called *Centistokes (cSt)*.

where,

1 *St* = 100 *cSt*

1 *cSt* = 10^{-6} m²/s

Since, the specific gravity of water at 68.4°F (20.2°C) is almost *one* (1).

For practical purposes, kinematic viscosity of water at 68.4 F is 1.0 Cst. Viscosity and temperature: For dynamic or kinematic viscosity, the reference temperature must be quoted as viscosity is highly temperature dependant. The kinematic viscosity decrease at higher temperature while in gas the kinematic viscosity increase at higher temperature. Other units of viscosity are Saybolt Universal Seconds (SUS) kinematic viscosity versus dynamic or absolute viscosity can be expressed as:

$$v = 4.63 \, \mu/SG$$

where,

  v = kinematic viscosity (SSU)
  μ = dynamic or absolute viscosity (cP)
SG = Specific Gravity

Degree engler: It is used as a scale to measure kinematic viscosity, in Great Britain. Unlike the Saybolt and Redwood scales, this scale is based on comparing a flow of the substance being tested to the flow of another substance, i.e. water. Viscosity in Engler degrees is the ratio of the time of a flow of 200 cm^3 of the fluid whose viscosity is being measured, to the time of flow of 200 cm^3 of water at the same temperature (mostly 20°C but sometimes 50°C or 100°C) in a standardized Engler viscosity meter (Table 1.2).

Table: 1.2: Viscosity and specific gravity of some common liquids

Centi stokes (cSt)	Typical liquid
1	Water (20°C)
4.3	Milk
15	Oil
20	Cream
43	Vegetable oil
220	Tomato juice
1100	Glycerine (20°C)
2200	Honey
6250	Mayonnaise
19,000	Sour cream

Viscosity and Temperature

It should be noted that for liquids viscosity decreases with temperature and for gases viscosity increases with temperature.

FLUID STATICS—MEASUREMENT OF PRESSURE

Pressure in Fluid and its Variation

Relationship between depth and pressure: When we dives under water surface, it is noticed that the pressure on ear drums is considerably higher than atmospheric pressure. For a given depth liquid exerts same pressure in all directions. The pressure of a liquid is directly proportional to the depth. As shown in Fig. 1.3, the fluid leave the tank at varying velocities. This is due to variation in pressure of fluid at different levels. Pressure is defined as the force per unit area. The force is due to the weight of the water above the point.

The pressure at any point of fluid increase with the depth. Down the column of a fluid, the increase in pressure is due to weight of fluid column above that level. To understand relation between pressure and depth of liquid column, consider a vertical column of liquid with constant cross-sectional area. It is assumed that the liquid is at rest (so no shear forces) and it is in equilibrium (all forces are balanced in the column).

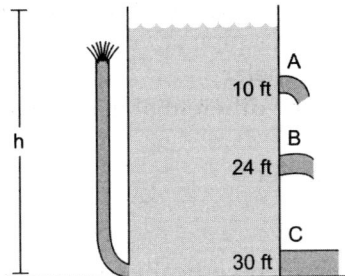

Fig. 1.3: Pressure versus depth

At any particular depth of the column, the weight of the column is balanced by force due to pressure at that point. Thus, the pressure at that point is equal to weight of column at that point divided by area of cross-section of liquid column.

Weight of column = Volume × Density × Acceleration due to gravity

Volume of liquid column = Height of column × Area of cross-section

Thus, pressure at any depth = Density of liquid × Acceleration due to gravity × Height of the liquid column above that point

In hydraulics, as per above equation as density and acceleration due to gravity are constant, the pressure varies with depth in liquid bodies.

The atmospheric pressure is the pressure acting on fluids over the surface of earth. The pressure measurement is done to find the weight of air column above the level. Thus, the absolute pressure in any fluid is equal to atmospheric pressure plus the pressure due to weight of fluid column above level of measurement. The pressure measured by pressure guages is the quantity in excess to the atmospheric pressure. The calibration of the pressure gauges are done, so that they indicate zero at atmospheric pressure.

Pressure reading above atmospheric pressure is positive and pressure reading below atmospheric pressure is negative. The pressure reading and difference of these devices from atmospheric pressure is known as guage pressure. The absolute pressure is equal to the sum of the guage pressure and the atmospheric pressure.

Pressure Measurement Devices

Different types of pressure measurement devices are available which ranges from simple gauges with low accuracy to complex gauges with high accuracy. Apart from this, other types of gauges are, gauges using fluids, gauges without fluids, electrical gauges, optical gauges and mechanical gauges.

A few commonly used pressure gauges are discussed below:
Manometer: It is a device used for measure the pressure of a fluid by balancing it with against a column of a liquid.

Classification of Manometer

I. **Simple manometers are** those which measure pressure at a point in a fluid contained in the pipe or a vessel. They are of many types:

a. Piezometer

b. U-tube manometer (simple manometer)

c. Single column manometer.

II. **Differential manometers** measure the difference of pressure between any two points in a fluid contained in a pipe or vessel. They are of following types:

    a. U-tube differential manometer

    b. Inclined or sloping U-tube differential manometer

    c. Micromanometer

    d. Inverted U-tube manometer.

I. Simple Manometers

a. Piezometer: It is a tube connected vertically to the liquid system which pressure is to be measured. The liquid rises in the tube up to the point, where the weight of the liquid column in the tube is balanced by the gauge pressure of the system. Pressure shown by the piezometer is the gauge pressure as the tube is open to the atmosphere on the other side as shown in Fig. 1.4.

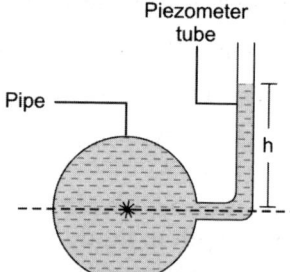

Fig. 1.4: Piezometer

Disadvantages

- It can measure gauge pressures only.
- It is not suitable for measuring negative pressures.
- They cannot be employed when large pressures in the lighter liquids are to be measured as this would require very long tubes that cannot be handled conveniently.
- Gas pressures cannot be measured by it.

    Note: These limitations can be overcome by the use of U-tube manometers.

b. U-tube manometer: It operates on the **principle of hydrostatic balance.** It is a U-shaped tube filled with an immiscible liquid, opens at both ends. In it, one end is attached to the fluid system and its pressure is to be measured whereas the other end is open to the atmosphere. At first, when the liquid enters the manometer the level of liquid is same in both the arms of manometer. As one arm of the manometer is under examination, the liquid falls in one arm and the level increases in the other arm. The gauge pressure of the system can be determined by the variation in the levels of the liquid as one of the ends is open to the atmosphere as it is shown in Fig. 1.5. For measuring high pressures a liquid used is heavy manometer, and for measuring low pressures liquid used is a light manometer.

    Depending upon the pressure of the source it measures, the liquid in the column of manometer will either increase or decrease when a manometer is attached to a process. Therefore, it becomes essential to have information about the type of the liquid and its height in the column in order to determine the pressure of the liquid. This is because the amount to which the level of the liquid will increase or decrease due to pressure depends on type of the liquid and also the specific gravity is important to measure the pressure correctly.

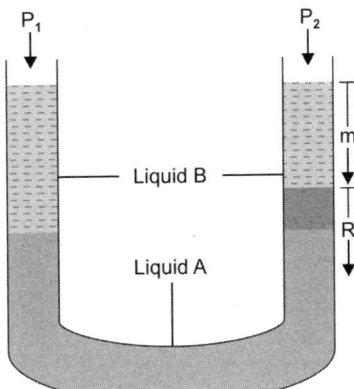

Fig. 1.5: U-tube manometer

The correctness of the manometer is influenced by the shape of liquid at the interface between the liquid and air in the column. This level of the liquid is known as meniscus and it varies with the shape of the liquid. Hence, the shape of the liquid can predict the type of the liquid that is being used.

In order to avoid the errors the shape of the liquid is determined at the centre of the column. The liquid should have the following characteristics:
- Low viscosity
- Low surface tension
- Non adherent to the walls of the container
- It should not evaporate
- The two liquids used should be immiscible.

The filled liquid must be clean and have a known specific gravity.

Advantages
- It is very simple in construction
- Cost-effective
- Accurate and sensitive
- Other process variables can be measured.

Disadvantages
- It is fragile in construction
- Shows too much sensitivity to temperature changes.

Applications
- Low pressure ranges can be calculated.
- It has extensive use in the laboratories.
- Venturi meter and orifice meter use it for flow determination.
- Calibration of gauges and various other instruments can be done.
- The fall of pressure in different valves and joints can be measured.

c. **Single column manometer:** It is a remodelled form of a U-tube manometer as shown in Fig. 1.6 which has a shallow reservoir attached to one end of the manometer. The shallow reservoir that is connected has a large cross-sectional area about 100 times in contrast to the area of the tube.

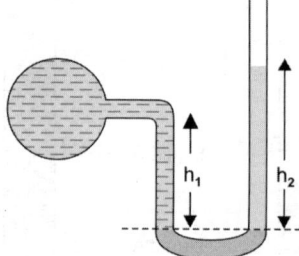

Fig. 1.6: Single column manometer

II. Differential Manometer

a. **U-tube differential manometer:** It is also called two-fluid U-tube manometer. It is also a U-tube manometer as shown in Fig. 1.7 having the two ends, connected to the two systems between which pressure difference is to be measured. It depends on the range of pressure differences, i.e. to be measured, a suitable liquid or combination of liquids can be filled in the two arms of the U-tube. If large pressure differences are to be measured a heavy manometer liquid is filled in the U-tube. And to measure very small pressure difference U-tube with long arms is used and two light liquids are filled in the two arms of the U-tube. It usually contains two immiscible liquids A and B having almost same densities.

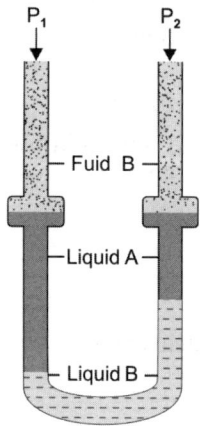

Fig. 1.7: Differential U-tube manometer

b. **Inclined or sloping U-tube manometer:** It is used for measuring the minute differences of two pressures (where accuracy is the major consideration). It is basically similar as differential U-tube manometer, but the tube is inclined at certain angle this time as shown in Fig. 1.8. The construction involves enlarged vertical leg so that due to movement of meniscus this enlargement becomes negligible. Although leg having meniscus is inclined in such a manner that for a small value 'r' it moves a considerable distance along the tube. It results in more deflection in the liquid level (in the tube) for the same change in pressure. Thus enables the measurement of small pressure changes with high accuracy.

c. **Micromanometer:** It is a different form of liquid column manometers. It is based on the inclined tube manometer and is useful in calculating the very small pressure

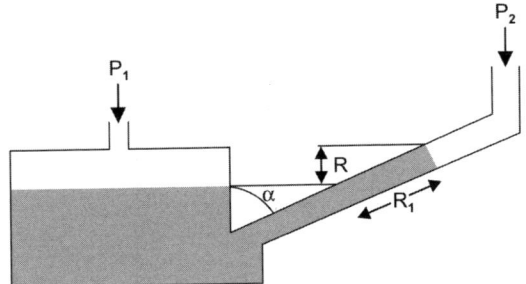

Fig. 1.8: Inclined manometer

variations. The meniscus of the inclined tube is at reference level as shown in Fig. 1.9, observed with a magnifier having a cross hair line. This is performed for the condition when $p_1 = p_2$ and the adjustment can be made by moving well high and low across a micrometer. Similarly, when p_1 is not equal to p_2 the well can be moved high and low to keep the meniscus at zero and the pressure can be measured by the difference between the two readings. Considering manometric fluid as a free body, the following forces are acting on it namely:

- Weight dispersion over the whole fluid.
- The drag force because of the movement of fluid and the resulting tube wall shearing stress.
- Force created because of differential pressure.
- Surface tension at both ends of manometer.

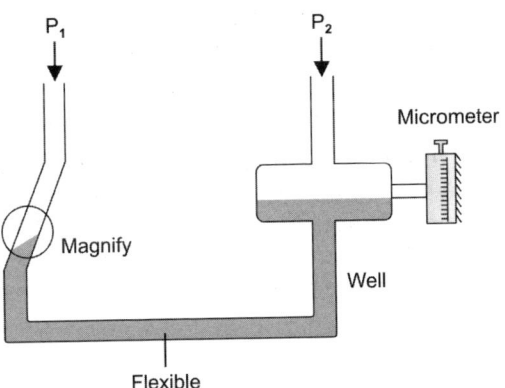

Fig. 1.9: Micromanometer

d. Inverted U-tube manometer: It is used when the difference between the densities of the two liquids is small. 'A' and 'B' are points at different levels with liquids having different specific gravity. It consists of a glass tube-shaped like an inverted letter 'U' and seems similar to two piezometers connected end-to-end to which air is present at the center of the two limbs as shown in Fig. 1.10. As the two points in consideration are at different pressures the liquid raises in the two limbs. Air or mercury is used as the manometric fluid.

2. Mechanical pressure measurement gauges: It involves the measurement of pressure with the help of a solid object like a tube, plate or diaphragm instead of measuring it by the deviation of fluid level in the tube. The object whose pressure has to be measured is attached to the deviating object. The change in the pressure deviates the object and

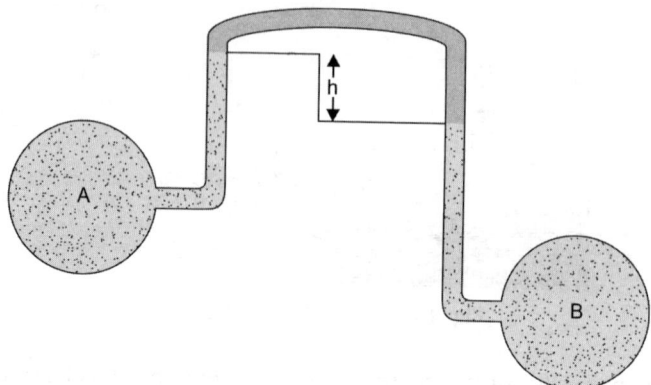

Fig. 1.10: Inverted U-tube manometer

the deviation produced is magnified with the help of a suitable gear and linkage mechanism and is depicted on the calibration dial.

3. Bourdon gauge: It involves a coiled tube in which one end is attached to the system and the other is sealed. The coil staighten up and results in the deviation of the sealed end by applying pressure in the tube.

The indicating needle is attached to the sealed end with the help of gear and linkage mechanism. The deviation produced at the sealed end leads to the movement of the needle on a calibrated dial. It is used to determine the wide ranges of pressure.

4. Diaphragm gauge: It resembles Bourdon gauge but it has a diaphragm that deviates when the pressure is changed and is depicted on calibrated scale.

5. Bellows gauge: This is used for determining very low pressures. In this gauge the indicating needle moves by the deviation of bellow chamber.

6. Pressure transducers: In this the pressure changes are converted into electrical signals with the help of a electrical system that is attached along with the mechanical gauges. They determines pressure continuously in a manner so that the electrical signals is delivered to some control system that can be used to determine the pressure changes. The types of pressure transducers are piezoelectric, magnetic, resistive, or capacitative.

FLUID DYNAMICS

The Bernoulli Equation

Daniel Bernoulli (1700–1782) was the first scientist who contributed in a fundamental way to the development of it. After Bernoulli, others who contributed to the development of the ideas were d' Alembert (1717–1783) but the theory was put on a firm foundation by the work of Euler (1707–1783). The conservation theorems which is closely related to the conservation of energy when applied to flow of fluids are collectively called Bernoulli theorems.

Bernoulli's theorem states that in an ideal flow state of an incompressible fluid the total energy per unit mass, which consists of pressure energy, kinetic energy and datum energy, at any point of fluid is constant.

Assuming a horizontal flow (neglecting minor elevation differences between measuring points) the Bernoulli equation can be modified to:

$$p_1 + 1/2 \, \rho \, v_1^2 = p_2 + 1/2 \, \rho \, v_2^2$$

where,

p = pressure
ρ = density
v = flow velocity

The equation can be adapted to vertical flow by adding elevation heights h_1 and h_2.

Assume a horizontal flow that neglects minor elevation differences between the measuring points and the Bernoulli equation then can be modified into:

$$p_1 + 1/2\, \rho\, v_1{}^2 = p_2 + 1/2\, \rho\, v_2{}^2$$

where,

p = pressure
ρ = density
v = flow velocity

The equation can be adapted to vertical flow by adding elevation heights h_1 and h_2.

Assuming a uniform velocity profiles in the upstream and downstream flow – then the continuity equation is expressed as:

$$q = v_1\, A_1 = v_2\, A_2$$

where,

q = flow rate
A = flow area

Combining these two equations and let assume $A_2 < A_1$, gives the "ideal" equation:

$$q = A_2\, [2(p_1-p_2)/\rho(1-(A_2/A_1)^2)]^{1/2}$$

For a given geometry (A), the flow rate can be known by measuring the difference in pressure $p_1 - p_2$.

The theoretical flow rate q will show smaller in practice be (2–40%) because of geometrical conditions.

The ideal equation can be changed with a discharge coefficient by:

$$q = c_d A_2\, [2(p_1-p_2)/\rho(1-(A_2/A_1)^2)]^{1/2}$$

where,

c_d = discharge coefficient

c_d (discharge coefficient) is a function of the jet size or orifice opening

$$\text{Area ratio} = A_{vc}/A_2$$

where,

A_{vc} = area in "vena contracta"

"Vena contracta" is explained as the minimum jet area which appears immediately to downstream of restriction. The viscous effect is usually expressed in terms of the Reynolds Number—Re which is a non-dimensional parameter.

In "Vena contracta" the velocity of the fluid will be highest and the pressure at the lowest due to the two equations Bernoulli and Continuity equation. The velocity will decrease to the similar extent after the metering device as before the obstruction. A head loss to the flow is added as the pressure recovers to a pressure level lowers than the pressure before the obstruction.

The above equation can be modified with diameters to:

$$q = c_d \pi/4\, D_2^2\, [2(p_1 - p_2)/\rho(1 - d^4)]^{1/2}$$

where,

D_2 = orifice, venturi or nozzle inside diameter

D_1 = upstream and downstream pipe diameter

$d = D_2/D_1$ diameter ratio

$\pi = 3.14$

The above equation can be convert into mass flow for fluids by just simply getting it multiply with density:

$$m = c_d \pi/4\, D_2^2\, \pi\, [2(p_1 - p_2)/\rho(1 - d^4)]^{1/2}$$

While measuring the mass flow in gases it is required to consider the pressure reduction and changes in density of the fluid. The formula above can be used for applications but with limitations that to bring relatively small changes in pressure and density.

Applications

- It is applied in the measurement of the rate of fluid flow using orifice meter, venturi meter, etc.
- It is applied in the working of centrifugal pumps
- It is easy to measure heights and apply them as energy terms.
- It can be used to calculate pressure or velocity of the fluid.
- It works in air flight and helps to fly by dragging against thrust force.

Types of Flow

Reynolds number is defined as the ratio between inertial and viscous forces and is denoted by Re. It is a well suitable parameter to determine whether the condition of flow is laminar or turbulent. It can be explained as when the viscous forces are dominant to keep all the fluid particles flow in line that is slow flow and low Re then the flow is termed laminar flow. The very low Re shows viscous motion and inertia effects are considered to be negligible. Similarly when the inertial forces are dominant over the viscous forces that is fast flow and high Re then the flow is termed turbulent flow.

It is a dimensionless number comprised of the physical characteristics of the flow. An increasing Reynolds number indicates an increasing turbulence of flow.

$$R = \frac{\rho V D}{\mu}$$

where,

V = velocity

D = distance

For example, as shown in Fig. 1.11 for fluid flowing in a pipe, V is the average fluid velocity, and D is the pipe diameter, excessive fluid inertia tends to disrupt organized flow leading to chaotic turbulent behaviour, whereas viscous stresses within a fluid tend to stabilize and organize the flow.

Reynolds numbers up to 2000 are laminar fluid flow. Reynolds number above 4000 is entirely turbulent flow. There is a transition in flow between laminar and turbulent in a range among 2000 and 4000, and makes possible to acquire sub-regions of both flow types within a flow field provided.

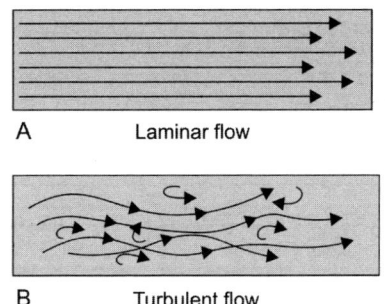

Figs 1.11A and B: A. Reynolds number equation; B. Laminar flow and turbulent flow

The fluid is governed by the laws of fluid statics when the flow is zero or it can be said statics.

Navier-Stokes equation is used in describing the laminar fluids flow and the Bernoulli equation is used to describe the viscous flow.

Significance

It is used to determine nature of flow, i.e. viscous or turbulent:

- Whether viscous/turbulent.
- It is helpful in determining the physical stability of suspensions or emulsions by studying type of flow.
- It is used to study the rate of heat transfer of liquids also depends on the flow.
- It is an important part in the calculation of the friction factor in equations of fluid mechanics, including the Darcy-Weisbach equation.
- It is used when modelling the movement of any organisms swimming through water.
- It is used to calculate atmospheric air which is considered to be a fluid and makes it possible to apply it in wind tunnel testing to study the aerodynamic properties of various surfaces.
- It also shows an important part in the testing of wind lift on aircraft, in cases of supersonic flights where the high speed causes a localized increase in the density of air surrounding the aircraft.

ENERGY LOSSES

Whenever a fluid is flowing through a pipe then the fluid experiences some resistance due to which some of the energy of the fluid is lost. The Bernoulli's equation includes the term energy losses in the pipe. Hence, it is very necessary to determine the energy losses. For the pipe system, the overall head loss of the head consists of loss due to viscous effects in the straight pipes and are termed the major loss and denoted $h_{L\text{-major}}$. The head loss in various others pipe components, termed the minor loss and denoted $h_{L\text{-minor}}$.

$$H_1 = h_{l\text{-major}} + h_{l\text{-minor}}$$

They are classified as in Fig. 1.12.

1. **Major energy losses:** The viscosity causes loss of energy in the flows which is known as frictional losses or major energy loss. The fluid flow can either be viscous or turbulent that influences losses. It can be calculated by:

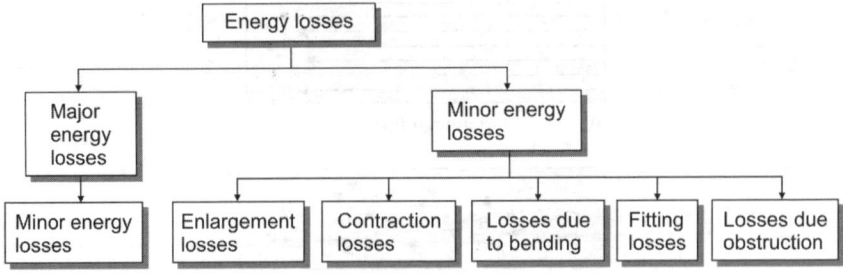

Fig. 1.12: Classification of energy losses

a. *The Darcy-weisbach formula*: It is valid for any fully developed, steady, incompressible pipe flow, whether the pipe is horizontal or on hill

$$h_f = 4fL\,V^2/(2gD)$$

where,

h_f = Loss of head due to friction

f = Co-efficient of friction which is a function of Reynolds number

$= 64/R_e$ (for Re < 2000) (laminar flow)

L = Length of pipe

V = Mean velocity of flow

D = Diameter of pipe

b. *Moody chart*: It is universally valid for all steady, fully developed, incompressible pipe flows.

The following equation from *Colebrook* is valid for the entire non-laminar range of the *Moody* chart. It is called *Colebrook formula*.

$$\frac{1}{f} = -2.0\log\left[\frac{\varepsilon/D}{3.7} + \frac{2.51}{\mathrm{Re}\sqrt{f}}\right]$$

c. *Fanning equation*: It is applicable when fluid is passing through a straight pipe and the nature of the fluid flow is viscous or turbulent. The roughness of the inner surface of the pipe is also a factor of consideration.

$$\Delta P_f = \frac{2f_{u^2}l\rho}{D}$$

where,

ρ = Density of the fluid

DP_f = Pressure drop

Friction losses can be reduced by the addition of soluble and high molecular weight polymers in a low concentration. Friction losses are permanent, since potential and kinetic energies are converted into heat.

2. **Minor energy losses:** The loss of energy due to change of velocity of the flowing fluid in magnitude or direction is called minor loss of energy. The minor loss of energy includes the following cases:

a. **Enlargement Losses:** Figure 1.13, the cross-section of the pipe enlarges gradually; the fluid adapts itself to the changed section without any disturbance

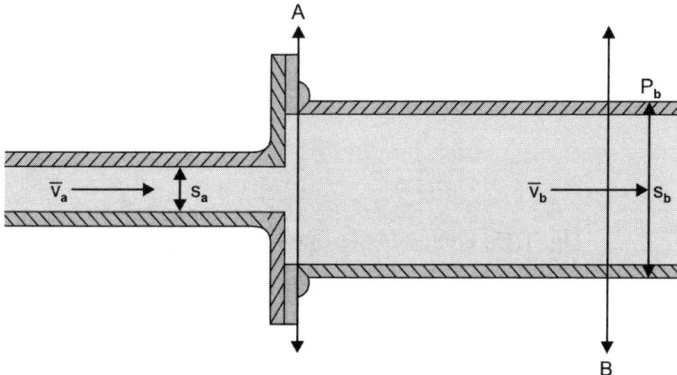

Fig. 1.13: Energy losses due to enlargement

resulting in loss of energy. But if the cross-section changes suddenly then loss of energy is seen due to eddies. Such disturbances causes loss of head.

The equation for head loss due to sudden expansion is:
$$he = (V_1 - V_2)^2/2\,g$$
where,

V_1 = The velocity at section 1
V_2 = The velocity at section 2

b. **Contraction losses:** (Figure 1.14) when the cross-section of the pipe is reduced at sudden the fluid flow becomes disturbed. The velocity of fluid at smaller cross-section known as vena-contracta will be far greater than that at larger section. The losses are observed due to additional eddying.

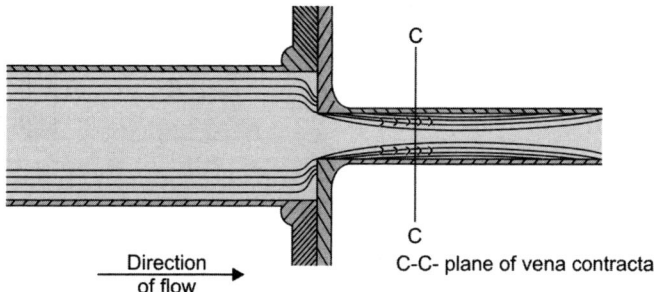

Direction
of flow   C-C- plane of vena contracta

Fig. 1.14: Energy losses due to contraction

The equation for head loss due to sudden contraction is
$$hc = k\,(V_2^2/2\,g)$$
where,

$k = ((1/C_c)-1)^2$
V_2 = The velocity at section 2

c. **Losses due to bending in pipe:** Change in direction causes fluid separation from the inner wall and a larger angle causes a greater head loss (Fig. 1.15). The radius of the bend and diameter of the pipe also contribute to the losses.

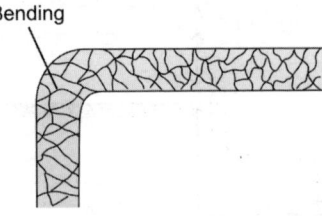

Fig. 1.15: Energy losses due to bending of pipe

The equation for head loss due to bending is

$$h_b = k \, (V^2/2 \, g)$$

where,

V = The velocity of the flow

k = The co-efficient of the bend, which depends on the angle of the bend, radius of curvature of bend and diameter of the pipe

d. Head loss due to pipe fittings: A large number of fittings are included in pipe, such as coupling, union, tee fitting, valve, elbow, etc. fittings causes disturbances in flow resulting in loss of energy causing head loss as shown in Fig. 1.16.

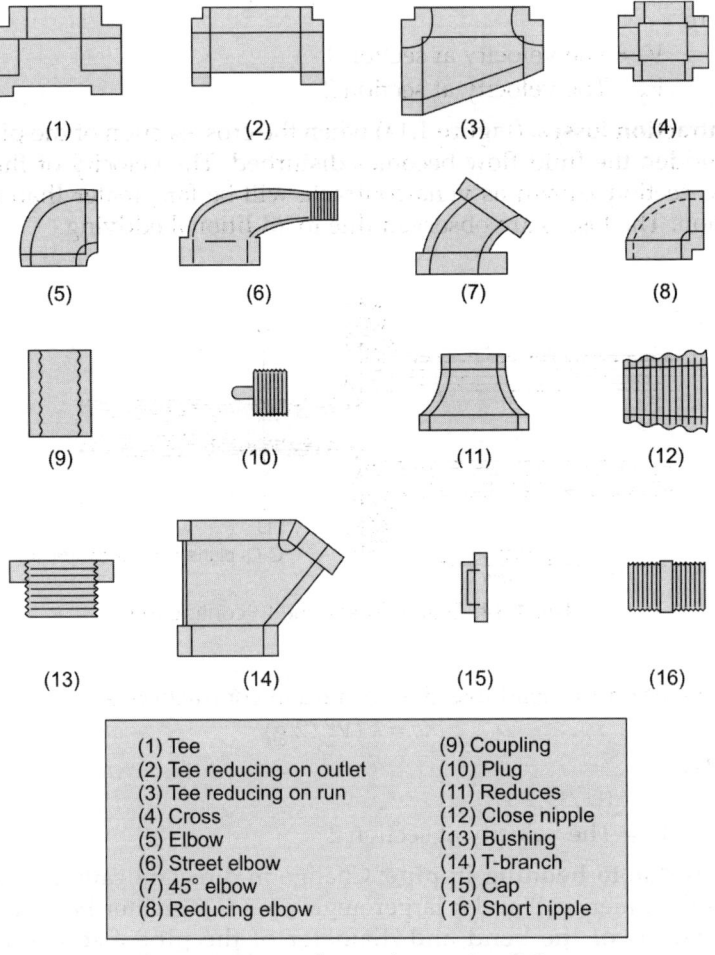

(1) Tee	(9) Coupling
(2) Tee reducing on outlet	(10) Plug
(3) Tee reducing on run	(11) Reduces
(4) Cross	(12) Close nipple
(5) Elbow	(13) Bushing
(6) Street elbow	(14) T-branch
(7) 45° elbow	(15) Cap
(8) Reducing elbow	(16) Short nipple

Fig. 1.16: Energy losses due to pipe fittings

The equation for head loss due to fitting losses is

$$h_f = K_L \, (V^2/2 \, g)$$

where,

V = The velocity of the flow

K = The coefficient of pipe fitting

Measures for Reducing Head Loss

- Replace pipes through the project lifetime by solids that will accumulate along the pipe walls, constricting the diameter and altering surface roughness
- Minimize pipe lengths and number of components as they both are directly proportional to head loss
- A uniform pipe diameter
- Operate at design velocity to reduce head loss.

Transportation of Fluids

Pipe, tubing, hose, fittings and accessories are used for the closed transfer of materials, typically liquids but also solids and gases. Pipes and tubes are often, but not always, cylindrical in shape. Products with a square cross-section are less common, but are also available. Pipes are designated mainly by their inner diameter (ID) while tubes are designated mainly by their outer diameter (OD). Hoses are flexible and often reinforced. Fittings and accessories are used to join pipes to pipes, pipes to tubes, or pipes to hoses.

Pipes and tubes may be used to transfer water and liquid chemicals, gases, such as propane and nitrogen, and solids, such as granular plastics and cereal grains. Although pipes are designated by ID and tubes are designated by OD, measured diameter is not the only distinction between the piping and tubing. Typically, pipes can withstand higher temperatures and higher pressures. Pipes are also used in closed systems with fittings, such as in a chemical processing facility. Tubes may be used with more open systems (e.g. drainage).

Measurement of flow of fluids: Flow measurement is required in many industries, e.g. oil industry, power plants, chemical industry, food and beverages industry, water and waste treatment plants. It is essential for determining the quantity of a fluid, gas, or steam, which passes through a check point, either through a closed conduit or by an open channel in daily processing operation. It is helpful in evaluation of volume, flow rate, mass flow rate, flow velocity, or other quantities.

The instrument that is used in measurement of flow is called flowmeter. The development of a flowmeter involves a wide variety such as flow sensors, the use of computation techniques in the sensor and fluid interactions, the signal processing units and the associated transducers, and in the assessment of an overall system in both the laboratory and the field under various conditions, such as ideal, disturbed, harsh, or potentially explosive.

Depiction of flowmeters: Flowmeters are integrated instruments that are used to measure the different flow quantities by using different technologies. Many features can be referred in categorizing the flowmeters. Flow metering mainly comprises of— orifice meter, venturi meter, nozzles flow, pitot tubes, positive displacement, turbine, vortex, electromagnetic, ultrasonic Doppler, etc.

In a flow metering device based on the Bernoulli equation the downstream pressure after an obstruction will be lower than the upstream pressure before. To understand orifice, nozzle and venturi meters it is therefore necessary to explore the Bernoulli equation.

THE ORIFICE METER

Principle: It consists of a thin plate containing a narrow and sharp aperture and when the fluid stream is allowed to pass through the narrow constriction, the velocity of the fluid increases as compared to upper stream resulting in the corresponding decrease in the pressure head. As it can be correlated by Bernoulli's theorem that the increase in velocity head with the decrease in pressure heads between two points that can be measured by manometer.

Construction

The orifice meter consists of a flat orifice plate made of stainless steel with a circular hole drilled in it as shown in Fig. 1.17. There are two pressure taps one at upstream from the orifice plate and another at just downstream. Generally, there are three methods of inserting the taps and the position of taps determines the coefficient of the meter. From face of orifice the tap location *1 inch* upstream and *1 inch* downstream is termed as Flange location. Similarly from face of orifice tap location 1 pipe diameter (actual inside) upstream and 0.3 to 0.8 pipe diameter downstream is called "*Vena Contracta*" location. And from face of orifice tap location 2.5 times nominal pipe diameter upstream and 8 times nominal pipe diameter downstream is a pipe location.

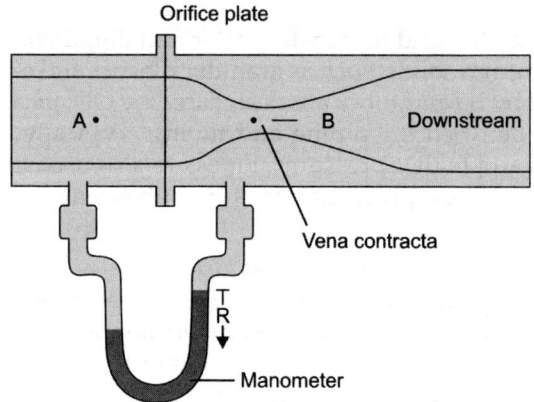

Fig. 1.17: Orifice meter

Working: It is used to the pressures across affixed constriction placed in the path of flow consisting of a constant area. According to Bernoulli's theorem, there must be a corresponding reduction in pressure at this point. The difference in pressure between the point of constriction and the main channel can be read using a manometer and this pressure difference can be related to the rate of flow of fluid. If manometer is connected to the Point A and B, the pressure at B will be less than at A and this pressure difference can be read from the manometer. If the two points A and B are chosen and Bernoulli's equation written between these two points:

The discharge coefficient—c_d—varies considerably with changes in area ratio and the Reynolds number. A discharge coefficient $c_d = 0.60$ may be taken as standard, but the value varies noticeably at low values of the Reynolds number. The pressure recovery is limited for an orifice plate and the permanent pressure loss depends primarily on the area ratio. For an area ratio of 0.5, the head loss is about 70–75% of the orifice differential.

Applications

- It has a wide applicability as it is standardized.
- Concentric orifice plates are used to measure flow rates of pure fluids.
- To measure flow rates of fluids containing suspended materials, such as solids, oil mixed with water and wet steam eccentric and segmental orifice plates are used.

Advantages

- The orifice meter is recommended for clean and dirty liquids and some slurry services.
- The rangeability is 4 to 1.
- The pressure loss is *medium*.
- Typical accuracy is 2 to 4% of full scale.
- The required upstream diameter is 10 to 30.
- The viscosity effect is *high*.
- The relative cost is *low*.

Disadvantages

- Poor pressure recovery at downstream
- Gets easily clogged when the suspended fluids flow
- Inaccuracy occurs as the orifice plate gets corroded
- The orifice plate has low physical strength
- Low coefficient of discharge.

The venturi meter: It is also known as restriction type flow meter. Its work is based on Bernoulli's principle. In it, pressure energy (PE) converted into kinetic energy (KE) to calculate flow rate (discharge) in a closed pipeline.

Principle: It consists of two tapered sections in the pipeline with a gradual constriction at its centre and when the fluid is allowed to pass through the narrow throat, the velocity of the fluid increases as compared to upper stream resulting in the corresponding decrease in the pressure head. As it can be correlated by Bernoulli's theorem that the increase in velocity head with the decrease in pressure heads between two points can be measured by manometer.

Construction: The venturi meter, as shown in Fig. 1.18, is usually made of cast iron, bronze or steel. The converging part is made shorter by employing large cone angle (19–21°) while diverging section is longer with lower cone angle (5–15°). The high-pressure tap is located at starting of the venturi and low-pressure tap located in the middle of throat sections that are inserted in the pipeline, with the tapers smooth enough and gradual enough so that there are no serious losses.

Working: In it the fluid is accelerated through a converging cone having an angle of 15–20°. The pressure difference between the throat and upstream side of the cone is measured and signal for the rate of flow is provided. Most of the kinetic energy is converted back to pressure energy as the fluid slows down in a cone with a smaller angle of 5–7°. No "Vena Contracta" is found because of the cone and a gradual reduction in the area. At the throat it is observed that flow area is at minimum. High pressure

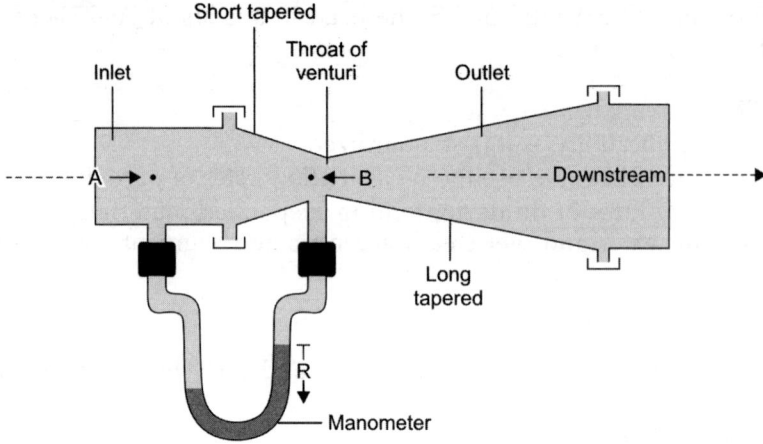

Fig. 1.18: Venturi meter

and energy recovery makes it very useful in cases where only small pressure heads are available.

As a standard discharge coefficient is $c_d = 0.975$, but this value fluctuates at low values of Reynolds number. In it pressure recovery is better than the orifice meter.

Applications

- It is used for measurement of fluids, gas, liquids, slurries, suspended oils and other processes
- It is also widely used in large diameter pipes such as in the waste treatment process
- They are suitable for measurement of dirty fluid as it allows solid particles flow through it because of their gradually sloping smooth design.

Advantages

- The venturi tube is suitable for clean, dirty and viscous liquid and some slurry services
- The rangeability is 4 to 1
- Pressure loss is low
- Typical accuracy is 1% of full range
- Required upstream pipe length 5 to 20 diameters
- Viscosity effect is high
- Relative cost is medium.

Disadvantages

- It is quite expensive
- Requires more space
- Ratio of throat diameter to pipe diameter cannot be changed
- Energy losses
- Impossible to clean out the pressure taps if they clog up with dirt or debris.

PITOT TUBE

Principle: It is also known as insertion meter. It consists of a sensing element with a small constriction as compared to the size of the flow channel. As the sensing element is inserted at the centre of stream there is increased in velocity of flow resulting in decrease in pressure head. Tube at right angles to the flow measures pressure head only whereas the tube that pointed upstream measures pressure head and velocity head. The difference in the readings above determines the velocity head.

Construction: The tubes are connected to the legs of a manometer in which one tube is perpendicular to the flow of direction and the other tube is connected parallel to the direction of flow. The size of the sensing element is very small as compared to the size of the flow channel.

Working: Suppose that two tubes be inserted as shown in Fig. 1.19. If the tube is right angles to the flow be properly designed, it will measure the pressure head only. The tube that points upstream will measure the pressure plus the velocity head. The reading R of the manometer will therefore measure the velocity head and

$$\Delta Hp = u^2/2 \text{ gc}$$

where,

ΔHp = The velocity head of the fluid corresponding to R.

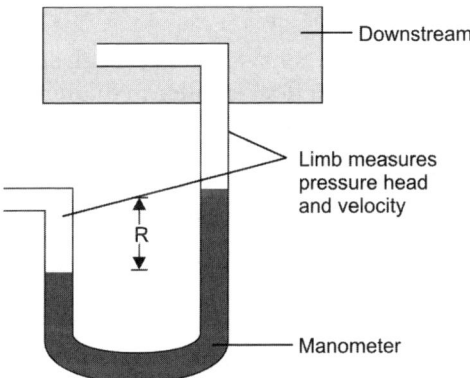

Fig. 1.19: Pitot tube

Whereas the orifice and venturimeter measure the average velocity of the whole stream of fluid, the pitot tube measures the velocity at one point only. Since, the velocity varies over the cross-section of the pipe, average velocity has to be calculated either from the maximum velocity or by taking reading at different points in the cross-section and determining the mean velocity by graphic integration.

Applications
- It is used in utility streams where high accuracy is not necessary
- It is also used in the air duct and pipe system
- It is used in aircraft for measuring the air flow velocity
- They can be used for mapping flow profile in a channel or duct.

Advantages
- Economical
- Minimum frictional loss
- Easy to install as having small size and in extreme environment, high temperature and pressure conditions

- Loss of pressure is negligible
- It measures the velocity at only one point.

Disadvantages

- Eddies within the pressure tube disturb the readings and creates more disturbances themselves
- It does not give average velocity
- It has low sensitivity and poor accuracy
- It is not suitable for dirty or sticky fluid like sewage disposal
- They can easily become clogged with foreign materials in the liquid.

ROTAMETER

The orifice and venturi meters depend on the measurement of a variable differential pressure across a fixed constriction placed in the flow. Since velocity varies with the pressure differential, these types sometimes referred to as "variable head" meters. In the rotameter, the area of flow is varied so as to produce a constant head differential, so it is also called "variable-area" meter.

Principle: A rotameter (Fig. 1.20) consists of a vertical, slightly tapered tube within which is placed a solid plummet or a float smaller in diameter than the narrowest part of the tube. As the flow of the liquid is increased or decreased, the plummet rises and falls freely, thereby varying the area of the annular space between it and the tube in such a way that head loss across this annulus is equal to the weight of plummet. The volumetric flow of the fluid may be directly read using the upper edge of the plummet as the index.

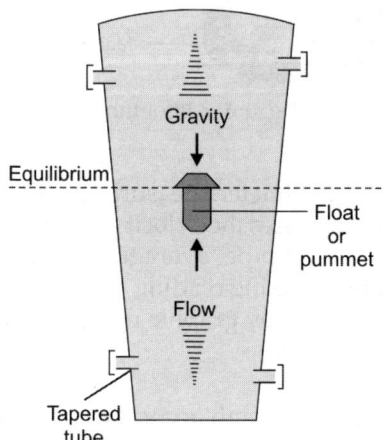

Fig. 1.20: Rotameter

Construction: It consists of a vertical shaped tapered tube, which is mounted with a narrow end down. The tube is usually made of glass and a nearly linear scale is etched and having solid plummet placed on a tube. The diameter of plummet is always smaller than the narrow end of the tube. Recording can be made by electric and electronic transmitters. Floats can be made of aluminium, lead, glass and plastic of different densities, so that a 200-fold range of flow can be measured accurately.

Working: The flow of fluid varies as the flow is upward through a tapered tube. The plummet which got surrounded by the fluid may rise and falls depending upon the rate of flow. The higher the plummet rises, the greater will be flow. In rotameters, the pressure drop is constant or nearly constant.

During the fluid flow, the area of the annular space between the plummet and the tube varies having an area is properly calibrated to the flow rate. These readings may be transmitted, for recording, integrating and controlling.

Applications

- It is used in chemical industries such as bulk drugs
- It has also been used in fermenters, the supply of air has controlled through it
- It is used both for gases and liquids at high and low pressures.

Advantages

- Direct visual readings
- Wide range
- Nearly linear scale
- Constant head loss
- It requires no straight pipe runs before and after the meters.

Disadvantages

- It will only be accurate for a given substance at a given temperature only.
- Resolution is relatively poor due to the direct flow indication.
- They are not generally manufactured in sizes greater than 6 inches/150 mm.

VERY SHORT QUESTIONS

1. Why is mercury used as a liquid in the manometer?
2. Write the following equations, explain its terms and mention its importance.
   a. Fanning equation
   b. Hagen-Poiseuille's equation
3. Briefly explain Reynold's number and its importance.
4. How is energy losses of energy due to enlargement in cross-section measured? Give relevant equation explaining all terms.
5. Define fluid mechanics and classify it.
6. Explain the fluid flow meter which gives point velocity.

SHORT QUESTIONS

1. Differentiate between fluid dynamics and fluid statics with suitable equation.
2. Compare and contrast the advantages and disadvantages of pitot tube and rotameter.
3. Explain types of fluid and the characteristic of different types of fluid.
4. What are merits and demerits of venturi meter over orifice meter?
5. Explain energy losses and mention essential measures to avoid it.

LONG QUESTIONS

1. Explain fluid and mention all relevant equations for calculation of flow rates.

2. Explain the working, principle, construction, advantages, disadvantages and uses of the following in detail:
   a. Venturimeter
   b. Pitot tube
   c. Orifice meter
   d. Rotometer

3. Elaborate energy losses that occur when a fluid flows throw a pipe with suitable equations.

4. Explain in detail Bernoulli's theorem and its significance.

5. Write a note on pressure measuring devices and explain working and principle of orifice meter.

MULTIPLE CHOICE QUESTIONS

1. The fluid flow in which the fluid particles in one layer do not mix with the fluid particles in the other layer is called:
   a. Laminar flow
   b. Turbulent flow
   c. Layer flow
   d. None of the above

2. Why is large reservoir used in single column manometer?
   a. In order to enhance the change in level of liquid in reservoir
   b. In order to negate the effects of change in level due to pressure variation
   c. In order to reduce the effect due to dynamic pressure variation due to motion
   d. None of the mentioned

3. Viscosity of a fluid can be defined as:
   a. Change in density of the fluid per unit temperature
   b. Flow resistance offered by the fluid
   c. Flow velocity change
   d. None of the above

4. Which of the following fluid can be considered as an ideal fluid?
   a. Viscous fluid
   b. Non-viscous fluid
   c. Compressible fluid
   d. All of the above

5. What is the SI unit for absolute or dynamic viscosity (μ)?
   a. Ns/m^2
   b. Nm^2/s
   c. N/m^2s
   d. N/m^2

6. Which of the following does not require manometer in the construction of flow of meters:
   a. Orifice meter
   b. Rotameter
   c. Venturimeter
   d. Pitot tube

7. **Venturi relation is one of applications of:**
   a. Equation of continuity
   b. Bernoulli's equation
   c. Light equation
   d. Speed equation

8. **If every particle of fluid has irregular flow, then flow is said to be:**
   a. Laminar flow
   b. Turbulent flow
   c. Fluid flow
   d. Both a and b

9. **The average drag coefficient for turbulent boundary layer flow past a thin plate is given by $C_f = 0.455/ (\log_{10} R_{el})^{2.58}$. Where R_{el} is the Reynolds number based on plate length. A plate 50 cm wide and 5 m long is kept parallel to the flow of water with free stream velocity 3 m/s. Calculate the drag force on both sides of the plate. For water, kinematic viscosity = 0.01 stokes:**
   a. 53.38 N
   b. 63.38 N
   c. 73.38 N
   d. 83.38 N

10. **Consider the above problem, estimate the value of Reynolds number:**
    a. 0.12
    b. 0.13
    c. 0.14
    d. 0.15

11. **The distance moved by liquid will be more in which type of manometer?**
    a. Inclined single column manometer
    b. Vertical single column manometer
    c. Horizontal single column manometer
    d. None of the mentioned

12. **Which device is popularly used for measuring difference of low pressure?**
    a. Inverted U-tube differential manometer
    b. U-tube differential manometer
    c. Inclined single column manometer
    d. Vertical single column manometer

13. **Which of the following uses direct reading of flow of fluids?**
    a. Orifice meter
    b. Rotameter
    c. Venturimeter
    d. Pitot tube

14. **What is kinematics viscosity of a fluid?**
    a. Dynamic viscosity per unit volume of the fluid
    b. Dynamic viscosity per unit weight of the fluid
    c. Dynamic viscosity per unit density of the fluid
    d. None of the above

15. **Generally, all the fluid particles in flowing fluid**
    a. Flow at a constant velocity
    b. Flow at various velocities
    c. Flow at a velocity as high as possible
    d. None of the above

Size Reduction

Mehfoozur Rehman and Yasmin Sultana

The term size reduction may be defined as the process of reducing the size of large solid materials of vegetables or chemical origin, to smaller units, coarse particles or fine particles. The process of size reduction is also known as diminution or pulverisation or comminution.

Polydispersed powders consists of different sized particles. So, they are termed polydispersed systems. These systems may create various problems in the production of dosage forms. Equal sized particles are ideal for pharmaceutical purpose. Powders with narrow size distribution can by pass the problems that encountered during the further processing.

Advantages

- Smaller and uniform particle size promotes the flow of the powder. It is advantageous for dye filling during the compression of tablets and also in hard gelatin capsule filling.
- Small and uniform sized particles can be rapidly and effectively dried as compared to larger sized particles.
- If the particle size is uniform and small, it will facilitate the mixing of ingredients. Smaller particles are more in numbers as compared to larger ones. This facilitates better mixing as well as content uniformity.
- Smaller particles effectively facilitate the rapid extraction and leaching of active ingredients from the tissue/cells of animals and plant origin because smaller particles allow rapid imbibition of solvents into it.
- Small particle size also improves the physical stability of suspension and emulsion by decreasing the rate of particle sedimentation.
- Size reduction increases the surface area, which facilitate the intimate contact of the solid particles with intestinal and/or gastric fluids. In this way dissolution rate increases.
- Size reduction also improves the rate of absorption because smaller particles absorb faster due to their enhanced dissolution rate. For example, sulphonamides shows their antibacterial activity at particle size of about 1 μm or less.

Disadvantages

- During the size reduction process drug may decomposed due to heat production. So, thermolabile substances are most affected.

- The substances that are less in particle size may be contaminated with the material used in construction of the grinding equipments, because during the grinding and milling process, the grinding surfaces may wear off. Such type of mills should be avoided, when drugs of high purity are required.

OBJECTIVES OF SIZE REDUCTION

The purpose of the size reduction are two:

- To produce smaller particles (e.g. to facilitate the mixing of powders or for the production of suspensions) or to increase the surface area (e.g. to increase adsorptive properties, to increase dissolution rate or to increase mass transfer coefficients).
- To crush or break apart minerals or crystals of chemical compounds which are intimately associated in the solid state.

MECHANISMS OF THE SIZE REDUCTION

Mechanisms of the size reduction depends on the nature of material, i.e. to be reduced. Generally, there are four main methods of size reduction that are described below:

- *Cutting:* In this type of mechanism materials are cut by means of a sharp blade, e.g. Cutter mill.
- *Compression:* In this method the material are reduced in size and are crushed by application of pressure, e.g. roller mill.
- *Impact:* In this mechanism of size reduction either material is less or more stationary which is hit by an object moving at high speed or the moving particles strikes a stationary surface, e.g. hammer mill.
- *Attrition:* In this method, size of the material is reduced by rubbing action between two relatively moving surfaces. The material is subjected to pressure such as in compression, e.g. fluid energy mill.

LAWS OF SIZE REDUCTION

There are number of theories that have been proposed to establish a relationship between energy input and the degree of size reduction produced.

Griffith theory: According to it, the amount of force to be applied on the crack length and focus of stress at the atomic bond of the crack apex. All solids contain flaws and microscopic cracks. A flaw in any structural weakness may develop into a crack under strain. The weakest flow in particle determines its fracture strength and controls the number of particles produced to largest possible pieces. This way the process continues until all flaws are fractured. It can be mathematically expressed as:

$$T = (Y_\varepsilon/c)^{1/2}$$

where,

T = Tensile strength

Y = Young's modulus

ε = Surface energy of the wall of crack

C = Critical crack path required for fracture

Rittinger's theory: According to it the energy required in a size reduction process is directly proportional to the new surface area produced.

$$E = K_R (S_n - S_i)$$

where,

E = Energy required for size reduction

K_R = Rittinger's constant

S_i = Initial specific surface area

S_n = Final specific surface area

Application: For size reducing of brittle materials that undergoes fine milling.

Bond's theory: According to it the energy used in crack propagation is proportional to the new crack length produced. The energy that has been used for deforming or fracturing a set of particles of equivalent shape is proportional to the changes in dimensions.

$$E = 2K_B (1/\sqrt{d_n} - 1/\sqrt{d_i})$$

where,

E = Energy required for size reduction

K_B = Bond's work index

d_i = Initial diameter of particles

d_n = Final diameter of particles

Application: It is useful in rough mill sizing. The work index is useful in comparing the efficiency of milling operations.

Kick's theory: According to it the energy used in deforming or fracturing a set of particles of equivalent shape is proportional to the ratio of change of size, or:

$$E = K_K \ln d_i/d_n$$

where,

E = Energy required for size reduction

K_K = Kick's constant

d_i = Initial diameter of particles

d_n = Final diameter of particles

Application: Kick's theory is mostly useful for crushing of large particles.

FACTORS AFFECTING SIZE REDUCTION

The use of wide variety of materials including chemical substances, animal tissues and vegetable drugs are widely employed in pharmaceutical industry. Therefore, there are numerous methods of size reduction. The properties affecting size reduction are:

• **Hardness:** It is the surface property of the material; an arbitrary scale of hardness has been developed, known as Moh's scale. According to this scale, substances of hardness up to 3 are known as soft; those between 3 to 7 are termed intermediate and above 7 are known as hard material.

• **Toughness:** Toughness is particularly encountered in fibrous material and it can be reduced by treating materials with liquefied gas (e.g. liquid nitrogen).

• **Abrasiveness:** It is the property which causes wear and tear of the grinding machine and contamination of the product.

• **Stickiness:** It causes adherence of materials to the size reduction machinery or choking of the meshes of the screen. For such type of materials, completely dry material is used or an inert substance is added during process.

- **Moisture content:** The percent of the moisture in the material affects the process of size reduction for dry grinding less than 5% of moisture is suitable and for wet grinding, more than 50% of moisture is suitable.
- **Softening temperature:** Size reduction process results in generation of heat which affects the waxy substances. In this case, the mill is cooled by circulation of water in surrounding water jacket.
- **Material structure:** Mineral substances have lines of weakness along which they splits to form flake like particles whereas vegetable drugs have a cellular structure.

EDGE RUNNER MILL

Principle: The size reduction mechanism is compression. Shearing force is also involved during the milling process.

Construction: It consists of two heavy rollers that may weigh several tonnes. The rollers move on a bed, which is made of stone or granite. Each roller has a central shaft and revolves on its axis. The rollers are mounted on a horizontal shaft and move around the bed as shown in Fig. 2.1.

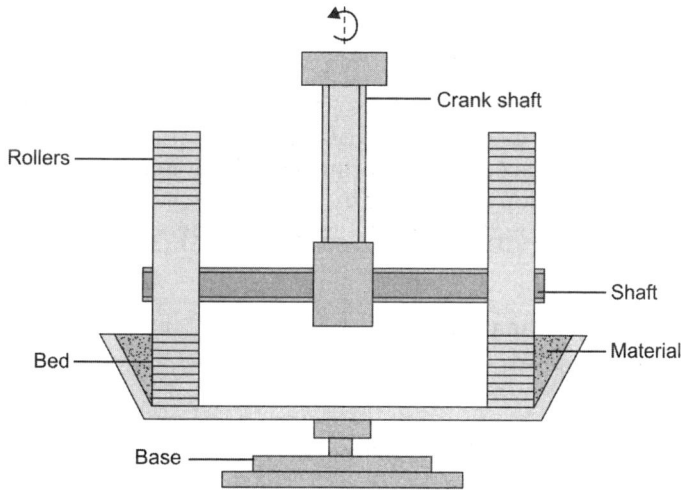

Fig. 2.1: Edge runner mill

Working: The material to be grounded is placed on the bed. With the help of a scrapper, it is kept in the path of the stone wheel. The stones revolve on its axis and at the same time interval around the shallow stone bed. The outer part of the wheel travel a greater distance than the inner and size reduction is achieved by shearing as well as crushing. The material is grounded for a definite period of time. The powder is collected and passed through a sieve to get powder of the required size. It is batch process.

Uses

- It is used for non sticky materials
- It can handle almost all drugs.

Advantages

- Edge runner mill is automatic no attention required
- It is used to produce fine materials.

Disadvantages

- It occupies more space than commonly used mills
- Contamination of the product is possible
- It is time consuming process
- It is not suitable for sticky materials
- High energy consumption.

END RUNNER MILL

Principle: The size reduction mechanism is compression due to heavy weight of steel pestle. It also involves shearing stress during the movement of mortar and pestle.

Construction: It is known as mechanical mortar and pestle as shown in Fig. 2.2. It consists of a steel mortar, which is fixed to a flanged plate. Underneath the flanged plate, a bevelled cog fitting is attached to a horizontal shaft bearing a pulley. Hence, the plate with mortar can be rotated at a high speed. The pestle is dumb-bell shaped so that balancing and efficient grinding by its weight can be achieved. The bottom of pestle is flat. The pestle carries an arm, which is hinged. By this arrangement, the pestle can be raised from the mortar to facilitate emptying and cleaning. The narrow central portion of the pestle is longer than the band of the arm around it. Hence, pestle can rise and fall over the material in the mortar.

Working: The material which has to be grounded is used to placed in the mortar. The scraper puts the material in the path of the pestle. The mortar revolves at a very high speed. The pestle is placed in the mortar. The revolving mortar leads the pestle to revolve and the size reduction is achieved by shearing as well as crushing. The material is collected and passed through a sieve to get the powder of desired size.

Uses

- It is used for non-sticky materials
- Almost all drugs are used.

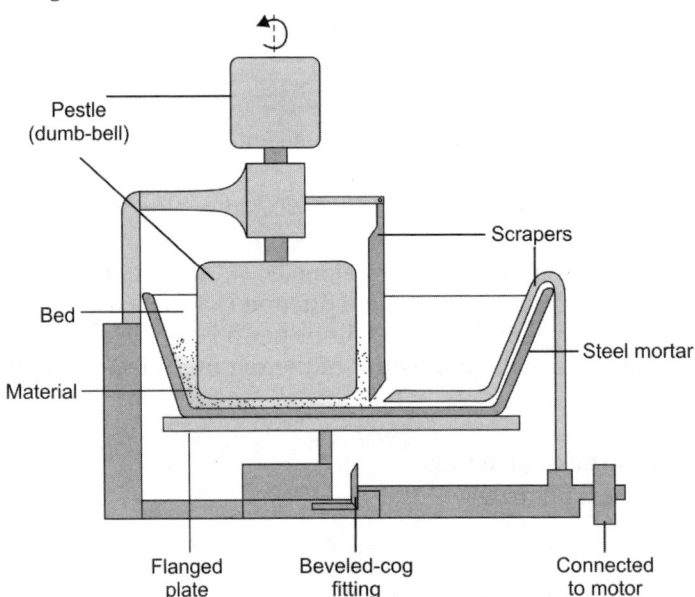

Fig. 2.2: End runner mill

Advantages
- It produces very fine particles
- It requires less attention during the milling operation.

Disadvantages
- Not suitable for drugs, which are in unbroken or slightly broken conditions and which are sticky in nature
- It is noisy.

Impact: The process of size reduction by using impact mechanism can be achieved by using hammer mill.

HAMMER MILL

Principle: The size reduction mechanism is impact occur between rapidly moving hammers which are mounted on a rotor and the powder material.

Construction: The hammer mill consists of four or more hammers that are attached to a central shaft, these hammer wing out to a radial position (Fig. 2.3). On the lower part of the casing there consists of a screen through which sufficient particle sized material can come out. The screen is made up of metal sheet and can be changed according to required particle size. Screens are even interchangeable to obtain fineness.

The shape of hammers may be of various types. It may includes: square-faced, tampered, cutting edged or stepped form. Hammers may be either rigid or swing type. Swing type hammers are more advantageous because it allows more clearance between hammers and screen. The interior of the casing may be smooth, circular or undulating in shape. The frequency of size reduction is more in undulating form casing due to repeated impacts as the particle is thrown back and forth between the hammer and the casing.

Working: The rotor operates at high frequency mostly up to 4800–5000 rpm. The speed of rotation depends on the diameter of the rotor which generally varies between 0.1 to 1 meter. The material is fed through hopper flowing vertically down and then horizontally and later in a circular motion. This beat the material to yield smaller particles which passes through screen giving considerably smaller size of materials than the aperture due to tangential exit.

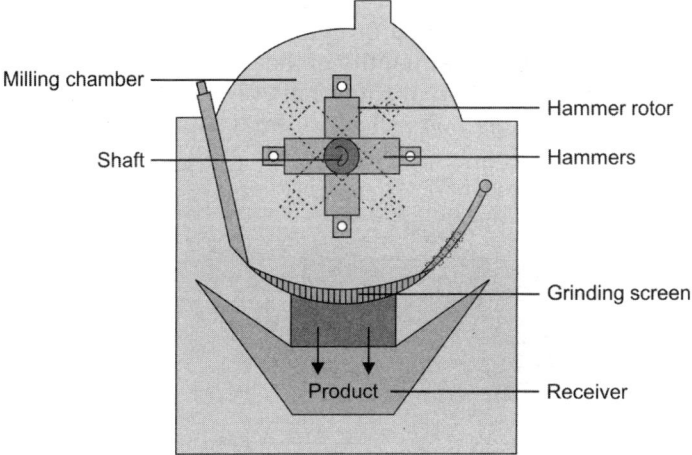

Fig. 2.3: Hammer mill

Uses
- Fine to moderate grinding of powders can be obtained
- Brittle material is best fractured by impact from blunt hammers
- Fibrous materials can be easily reduced to desired reduction by cutting edges.

Advantages
- Rapid in action
- Capable of grinding many different types of materials
- There are little chances of contamination of the product with abraded metal
- It is operated in a closed environment
- The process of size reduction is easily controllable.

Disadvantages
- It cannot be employed to reduce the size of thermolabile, fibrous, sticky and hard materials
- The rate of feeding should be controlled otherwise mill may choked
- Mill cannot be employed for abrasive materials.

COMBINED IMPACT AND ATTRITION

Ball Mill

Ball mill is also known as tumbling mills or pebble mill.

Principle: It works on the principle of both impact and attrition. The rapidly moving balls and the powder both are enclosed in a hollow cylinder, and at low speeds the ball rolls over each other and predominant mode of action will be attrition.

Construction

Ball mill consists of a hollow cylinder made of a metal and is lined with chrome, porcelain or rubber (Fig. 2.4). Cylinder is mounted on a metallic frame and can be rotated on its longitudinal axis. The length of the cylinder is more than its diameter. The cylinder contains balls that occupy about 30–50% of the volume of mill. These balls acts as grinding medium. The balls are made of steel, stoneware, iron or rubber. The size of the ball depends on the size or amount of the material that is to be reduced in size. The shape of the balls that are commonly used for pharmaceutical purpose, may includes round ball, cube shaped or cylindrical. The material to be reduced in size is placed into the cylinder. The quantity of the material that is filled in the cylinder should not exceed more than 60% of the internal volume. A constant numbers of balls are placed and the mill is rotated on its longitudinal axis.

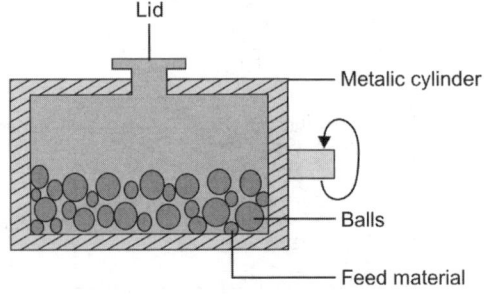

Fig. 2.4: Ball mill

Working: For the efficient size reduction, the rotation speed of the cylinder should be optimum. At slow speed the ball roll over each other, at this speed mechanism of the attrition will work for size reduction. This type of speed is used for wet grinding. At high speed, due to the centrifugal force balls are sticked on the mill wall and goes nearly to the top of the mill and then they fall to the bottom for recycling the process. At higher speed, due to centrifugal force, the balls are thrown out of the wall of the mill, due to this grinding of the materials will not takes place (Fig. 2.5). At critical speed, the centrifugal force just occurs, as a result the balls are picked up by the mill wall and carried nearly to the top from there they break contact with the wall and fall to the bottom. Thus, impact stress is also induced and the size reduction is made effective.

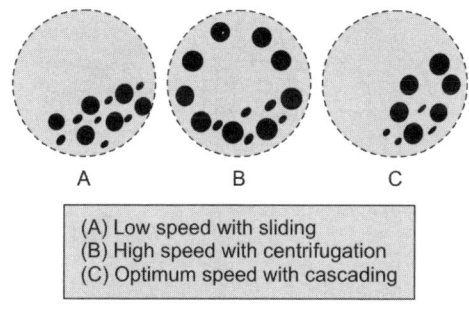

(A) Low speed with sliding
(B) High speed with centrifugation
(C) Optimum speed with cascading

Fig. 2.5: Ball mill operation

Uses
- Used for the final grinding of drugs and also for grinding suspensions
- Also used for milling ores prior to manufacture of pharmaceutical chemicals.

Advantages
- It helps to produce very fine powder (particle size ≤10 microns)
- It is suitable for milling toxic materials since it can be used in a completely enclosed form
- It has a wide application
- It is used for continuous operation
- It is used in milling of highly abrasive materials.

Disadvantages
- Contamination of product may occur as a result of wear and tear which occurs principally from the balls and partially from the casing
- High machine noise level especially if the hollow cylinder is of metal, but can be minimised by use of rubber
- Time consuming
- It is difficult to clean the machine after use.

FLUID ENERGY MILL
Fluid energy mill is also known as jet mill, micronizers or ultrafine grinders.

Principle: It operates on principle of impact and attrition. Material, i.e. to be reduced in size is suspended in a high velocity air stream. Particles are reduced due to high velocity collision between the suspended particles.

Construction: Fluid energy mill is constructed with an elliptical pipe made of either stainless steel or ceramics. The height of the pipe is about 2 meters and diameter may be ranging from 0.2 to 2 meters. The surface of the mill can be easily removed or replaced, if they are excessively eroded after being used. About two to six nozzles are also tangentially placed at the bottom of the elliptical pipe. A venture feeder also attached in the path of airflow. A cyclone separator which also acts as outlet is fitted to allow escape of air (Fig. 2.6).

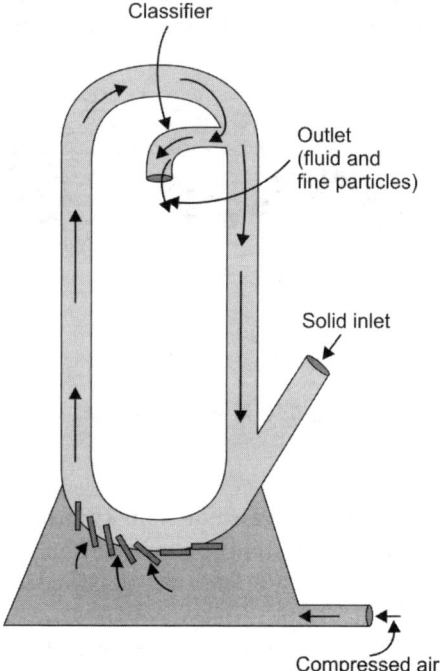

Fig. 2.6: Fluid energy mill

Working: The material that is to be reduced in size is introduced through the inlet. The composed air (used at 600 K pascal to 1 M pascal) entering through fluid nozzles transport the powder in the circular track of elliptical pipe. Due to the turbulent stream flow of air, the suspended particles collide with each other and get reduced in size. Then the smaller particles are carried to outlet and removed by cyclone separator. The larger particles re-circulated in the circular chamber and collide again to each other. And product is collected via sieve or in a bag collector which is further carried to size separation.

Uses
- To achieve ultra fine particles of the drugs, such as antibiotics and vitamins
- Very fine size can be obtained
- High and desirable quality control can be achieved
- Moderately hard materials can be used
- It is the first choice of mill when higher degree of drug purity is required
- It is used in milling of thermolabile materials.

Advantages

- It can be used to reduce the particle size of heat labile substances
- Ultra fine particles ($\leq$ 30 µm) can be achieved by this method
- Chances of contamination are negligible
- The machine has no moving parts and thus, the tendency of contamination due to wear parts is minimized
- The equipment is easily sterilized.

Disadvantages

1. It is an expensive process.
2. Fibrous, soft and tacky materials can be milled by using fluid energy mill.
3. Tendency of forming aggregates or agglomerates after milling.

ENERGY AND POWER REQUIREMENT FOR MILLING

In the process of size reduction, materials are reduced in size by breaking them. Firstly, material is crunched by the action of mechanically moving parts of the milling machine and as strain energy prevail beyond a limit, i.e. a function of the material fracture occurs along the line of weakness and there is release of stored energy.

Milling is obtained by mechanical stress then followed by rupture and the energy required depends upon the hardness of the material and also on the other specific properties of the material.

The forces applied to reduce size of material may be compression, impact or shear forces. In order to achieve efficient grinding, the energy applied to the material should be the minimum energy required to rupture the material. The studies of important factors in the process of size reduction are the amount of new surface formed by grinding and the amount of energy used. The basic assumption on which the milling depends upon is that the energy required to produce a change dL in a particle of size dimension L is function of L:

$$dE/dL = KL^n$$

where,

dE = Differential energy required

dL = Change in a dimension

L = Magnitude of a typical length dimension and K and n are constant

Kick states that the energy required to reduce a material is directly proportional to the size reduction ratio dl/L

$$K = K_k f_c$$

where,

K_k = Kick's constant and

f_c = Called the crushing strength of the material, which is given by the following equation:

$$dE/dL = K_k f_c L^{-1}$$

which on integration gives:

$$E = K_k f_c \log_e (L_1/L_2)$$

This equation states the Kick's law.

According to Rittinger the energy required for size reduction is directly proportional to the change in surface area.

$$K = K_R fc$$

therefore,

$$dE/dL = K_k f_c L^{-2}$$

where, K_R is called Rittinger's constant, and integration of the above equation gives: $E = K_R fc (1/L_2 - 1/L_1)$ this equation is known as Rittinger's law.

This bond states that energy used for deformation or fracturing the particle of equivalent shape is proportional to the change in particle dimension. Bond postulation is given by the following equation:

$$E = E_i (100/L_2)^{1/2} [1-(1/q^{1/2})]$$

In Bond's equation, if L is expressed in microns. E_i is defined as Bond's work index, which is the work required to reduce a unit weight from a theoretical infinite size to 80% which can pass through 100 μm sieve. These equations are used in making comparisons between power requirements for various degree of reduction.

SIZE REDUCTION IN PHARMACEUTICALS AND IN NANOTECHNOLOGICAL BIOMEDICAL PRODUCTS

Nanomaterials are superior materials which exhibits the characteristics at the size range of 1–100 nm. It can be made with a variety of chemical compositions, their surface can be tuned with various functionalization group on it, which ultimately leads to various characteristics features. As far as due to small size of nanomaterials, which exploited in drug delivery applications via possessing of unique properties. In the drug delivery aspects, nano size range exhibits enhanced permeation, absorption through gastrointestinal tract and enhanced permeation and retention effects by other absorption sites too. Moreover, the outer surface of nanomaterials can be tuned up with various molecular structures, which results to enhance circulation time passive targeting and active drug targeting.

Another aspects of nanomaterials in drug delivery is to encapsulates a variety of drug molecules, i.e. hydrophilic and hydrophobic drugs as its according to solubility of drugs. Therefore, day-to-day, the demand of nanomaterials is increasing in drug delivery and drug targeting area for treatment of different diseases by facilitating of sustained release, higher drug concentration at the desired sites and minimizing of the side effects, which resulted to better pharmacokinetics and pharmacodynamics effects.

Nanoparticles of defined size and chemical composition are required for various pharmaceutical applications. In recent advances in aerosol science and technology synthesizing nanoparticles, which have great potential for up and out scaling. Drug loaded nanoparticles through aerosols based delivery can be delivered efficiently to different parts of the human body. Other nanoparticles like magneto pharmaceuticals can be administered to the human body for diagnostics and imaging action. Another application of nanoparticles is biodetection of pathogens, tumor destruction via heating, tissue engineering and localized treatment such as hyperthermia.

Nanodermatology is fast growing application of nanomaterials in topical diseases. Nano scaffolds wound dressing exhibits superior therapeutic action for settlement of infectious, non-infectious, inflammatory disorders, wound healing and skin cancer. Nanoemulsions and nanopigments have been utilized in cosmetics in prevention of skin damage and maintains skin tone. Another application is quantum dots which impart a function in diagnostics in the detection of skin neoplasm.

VERY SHORT QUESTIONS

1. Explain the necessity of sieve in the size reduction equipment.
2. Why screen types of sieves gives more fine powders than the wire woven sieves?
3. Differentiate between:
   a. Dry and wet grinding.
   b. Mechanisms of attrition and impact.
4. Explain why there is a requirement of so many types of mills.
5. What is the affect of stickiness in the process of size reduction?
6. How size reduction of a material enhances the action of drugs?

SHORT QUESTIONS

1. Explain the principle, construction and uses of mill used for fibrous material.
2. Define size reduction and explain its objectives, advantages and disadvantages.
3. Explain the theories related to the size reduction of a powder.
4. Describe aseptic grinding process of antibiotics.
5. Explain the principle, construction and applications of mill used for thermolabile drugs.
6. What are energy requirement for size reduction?

LONG QUESTIONS

1. State the factors affecting size reduction.
2. Explain the principle, construction, working, uses, advantages and disadvantages of the following:
   a. Ball mill
   b. Hammer mill
   c. Fluid energy mill
   d. Edge runner mill and end runner mill.
3. What is ultra-fine grinder? Explain the construction, working, advantages and disadvantages of ultra-fine grinder.
4. Describes the law governing size reduction.
5. Explain the mechanisms and modes related to the size reduction of a powder.

MULTIPLE CHOICE QUESTIONS

1. Principle of colloid mill is based on the:
   a. Attrition
   b. Impact
   c. Shearing
   d. Compression

2. **The nature of pharmaceutical powders is:**
   a. Monodisperse
   b. Polydisperse
   c. Bidisperse
   d. None

3. **Size reduction application is:**
   a. Physical stability
   b. Dissolution rate
   c. Rate of absorption
   d. All of the above

4. **Size reduction in solid has mode of stress:**
   a. Impact
   b. Attrition
   c. Compression
   d. All of the above

5. **Mill used for hygroscopic materials is:**
   a. Colloid mill
   b. Percolation ball mill
   c. Fluid energy mill
   d. Hammer mill

6. **Type of metal used for making the sieve:**
   a. Zinc
   b. Stainless steel
   c. Tin
   d. Aluminium

7. **The principle of hammer mill:**
   a. Impact
   b. Attrition
   c. Compression
   d. Cutting

8. **According to IP 1996 the pharmaceutical powders were classified into how many types?**
   a. 3
   b. 4
   c. 5
   d. 6

9. **The principle of ball mill is:**
   a. Impact
   b. Attrition
   c. Both a and b
   d. None

10. **Most commonly used size reduction instrument in laboratory is:**
    a. Ball mill
    b. Hammer mill
    c. Colloid mill
    d. None of the above

11. **Principle of fluid energy mill:**
    a. Impact
    b. Attrition
    c. Both a and b
    d. None of the above

12. **Principle of hammer mill is:**
    a. Impact
    b. Attrition
    c. Both a and b
    d. None

13. **Principle of crushers is:**
    a. Impact
    b. Attrition
    c. Compression
    d. None

14. **In motor and pestle, the material is crushed by the application of:**
    a. Attrition and pressure
    b. Impact and attrition

    c. Attrition and cutting

    d. Impact and compression

15. **Edge runner mill acts on the principle of:**
    a. Compression
    b. Attrition
    c. Impact
    d. None

16. **Which of the following is not involved in a mode of stress applied in size reduction?**
    a. Cutting
    b. Compression
    c. Impact and attrition
    d. None

17. **Which of the following is not an example of grinders?**
    a. Roller mill
    b. Hammer mill
    c. Ball mill
    d. Fluid energy mill

18. **Fluid energy mill is an example of:**
    a. Crusher
    b. Grinder
    c. Ultrafine grinder
    d. Cutting machine

19. **Commonly used balls in ball mill are:**
    a. Round ball
    b. Banded ball
    c. Cube ball
    d. All of the above

20. **The following is not considered as a factor on selection of particular equipment for size reduction:**
    a. Feed and milled product
    b. Safety and economics
    c. Both a and b
    d. None

21. **Which equipment is suitable for crush soft tissue to help in the penetration of solvent during extraction process?**
    a. Hammer mill
    b. Ball mill
    c. Roller mill
    d. Fluid energy mill

22. **Which size reduction techniques is used for preparing suspension, emulsion and ointments?**
    a. Roller mill
    b. Fluid energy mill
    c. Colloidal mill
    d. Ball mill

23. **For brittle drug, which equipment is suitable for size reduction?**
    a. Cutter mill
    b. Ball mill
    c. Roller mill
    d. Fluid energy mill

Size Separation

Iram Khan and Yasmin Sultana

Sieving is also known as size separation, sifting, classification or screening. This is based on physical differences between the particles, such as size, shape, and density. It is a method of separating particles according to their size only. Particles can be separated into individual size by sieving. The material that remains on the given screening surface is known as oversize and the material that passing through the screening surface is known as undersize material.

OBJECTIVES

- It is applicable to formulate a uniform dosage form
- For preparation of granules of required size
- For separation of undesirable particles.

Applications

- Size-reduced particles are often passed through sieves to get fractions of narrow size range as all solid materials do not give a same size after size reduction and contains particles of varying sizes
- To avoid weight variation during tablet granulation the granules should be within narrow size range during tablet punching
- As a method determine particle size distribution, that may be useful for the preparation of capsules
- As a quality improving tool to analyse the raw materials, such as aspirin, griseofulvin, etc.
- It is employed to optimise the process condition, such as time of screening, feed rate, method of agitation, etc.
- Helps in recovering products from by products
- Helps in preventing and controlling environmental pollution
- It is widely applicable to control the emission of pollutants in power plants, steel mills, pharmaceutical producers, food manufacturers, chemical producers or other industrial companies.

OFFICIAL STANDARDS FOR POWDERS

Indian pharmacopoeia has prescribed standards for powder for pharmaceutical purpose. Degree of coarseness and fineness is expressed with reference to through which powder is able to pass, i.e. the nominal aperture size of sieve. The powders grades, sieve number, nominal aperture size are given in Table 3.1.

Coarse Powder

All the particles of powder that pass through a sieve with nominal mesh aperture of 1.7 mm (which is sieve number 10) and not more than 40% through a sieve with nominal aperture of 355 μm (which is sieve number 44) is known for coarse powder. Similarly other definitions can be written for the contents of the Table 3.1.

Sieving

The most frequently used method for size separation is sieving. They are constructed as a wire cloth with square shape meshes, woven by wire of brass, bronze, stainless steel or any desired material. Sieve should not be coated or plated. There must be no reaction between the material of the sieve and the substances that are to be sieved. Mostly sieves used are of kind of wire mesh type, the number of the sieve indicates the number of meshes found in a length of one inch in each direction parallel to the sieves. It should be very clear that it is the number of meshes that is required to be specified and not the number of wires. By this way we can conclude that a number 10 sieve has 10 meshes per inch in each direction, but it must be very clear that if there were 10 wires then there would be 9 meshes only. The size of the particles that will pass through the sieve will depend on the diameter of the wire (Table 3.1).

Table 3.1: Grades of powders and sieve no. along with aperture size as per IP

S. No.	Powders grades	Sieve number	Nominal mesh aperture size (mm)	Sieve through which 40% particles pass	Nominal mesh aperture size (μm)
1	Coarse	10	1.7	44	355
2	Moderately coarse	22	710	60	250
3	Moderately fine	44	355	8	180
4	Fine	85	180	–	–
5	Very fine	120	125	–	–

STANDARD FOR SIEVES

It is required that wire-mesh sieves should be made of uniform wire having circular cross-section for each sieve. The following particulars are stated as:

Numbers of sieve: They are a number of meshes in a length of 1 inch in each direction that is parallel to the wire.

Nominal size of aperture: It represents the length of the side of the square aperture so, it is the distance between the wires.

Nominal diameter of the wire: Nominal diameter of the wire and the number of meshes forms the basic standards for the sieve. The diameter of a wire is selected to give a suitable aperture size.

Approximate percentage of sieving area: It is standard which expresses the area of the mesh as a percentage of the total area of the sieve which depends on the size of the wire that is used for any particular sieve. Therefore, the sieving area is kept within the range of 35 to 40% so as to obtain suitable strength to the sieve.

Aperture tolerance average size: A few changes in the aperture size are unavoidable and are expressed as a percentage that is called the aperture tolerance average. As per IP it has a limit within which a particular dimension or aperture size are allowed to vary and can be acceptable for the purpose for which it can be utilised. An aperture tolerance average size is higher for fine sieves than the coarse sieves.

Material Used for the Construction of Sieves

For the construction of sieves officially, it is stated that there should be uniformity in wire circular cross-section. The material must have desirable strength in order to avoid distortion and be resistant to corrosion by any substances that are to be sieved. The wires of sieves are constructed by metals and non-metals.

Metals

Iron: Although iron is very cheap material for the construction of wires but it is very prone to rusting and it may contaminate the products.

Coated iron for: The protection from corrosion the iron may be coated by galvanising or tinning.

Copper: It is the commonly used material having the advantage of avoiding the risk of iron contamination. It is a soft material and meshes can be distorted easily.

Stainless steel: It is most expensive material for the construction of wires. It is the most satisfactory material, having resistance to corrosion.

Non-metals

Materials of natural origin, like—hair, silk, synthetic fibres-nylon, terylene are used in the manufacturing for wires. They have considerable strength and resistance to corrosion.

Methods of Size Separation (Sieving Methods)

There are various sieving methods that are discussed below:

Mechanical Sieving Methods

These methods are based on agitation or brushing the sieve or by using centrifugal force.

Agitation Method

Sieves can be agitated by different way:

Oscillation: In this method sieves are mounted on a frame and are oscillated to and forth. This is considered as a simple method but found that material may roll on the surface of the sieve and tend to acquire ball like shape particularly of fibrous materials.

Vibration: In this method mesh is vibrated electronically, at high speed. Due to rapid vibration of the particles, there is very less chance of binding of mesh.

Gyration: In this method sieves are placed on a rubber mounting and connected to an eccentric flywheel. The sieve is given rotator movement of small amplitude with suitable intensity. It provides spinning motion to the particles.

Brushing Methods

In this type of sieving method brush helps to move particles on the surface of the sieve and also used for cleaning of the sieve.

Centrifugal Methods

In this normally a vertical cylindrical sieve is used with a high speed rotor inside the cylinder so, that the particles are thrown outside by centrifugal force.

Wet Sieving

In this method particles are suspended in liquid and passes through the sieve with less binding of the sieve.

Fluid Classification

Industrial method of particle size separation may be based on sedimentation or on elutriation.

Size Separation Equipment

They are classified as:
- Sieving, e.g.
  - *Grizzles*: For coarse materials above 50 mm—large lumps
  - *Revolving screens*: Separations above 13 mm—trammels
  - *Shaking screens*: Separations from 13 mm downwards to fines
  - *Vibrating screens*: Coarse size 13 mm to fines
  - *Oscillating screens*: Fine mesh size
  - *Fluidized systems*: For very fine powders
- *Sedimentation*, e.g. sedimentation tank
- *Elutriation method*, e.g. double cone classifier
- *Centrifugal separation*, e.g. cyclone separator, air separator
- *Filtration*, e.g. bag filter.

Selection of Size Separation Equipment

The size separation equipment can be selected on feed material, nature of finished products, facilities available, cost in terms of procurement and maintenance. The most efficient method should be selected on particle properties.
- If particles are already present in suspension as obtained from colloidal mill or fluid energy mill then separation can be achieved by elutriation and cyclone separation
- As there are many pharmaceuticals solids which are water soluble, separation must be restricted to the use of air or sieve methods.

Sedimentation

Methods involving variations in the rates of settling of particles of various sizes and materials either when particles are too small to be screened effectively or large quantities of material required to be handled. For example, if two dissimilar particles having varying settling rates in water are kept in an upward flowing flow and the velocity of water is regulated so, it may lies between the settling rates of the two particles, and settling particles will move downward against the water flow to achieved separation.

Similarly another example if there are two particles having different settling rates introduced horizontally into water containing tank. It is observed that both the particles start settling. The rapid settling particle reaches the bottom of the tank first while the slower moving particle later. It can be seen that the settling rate of a particle depends on density, size and shapes.

Hence above described procedures are called classification methods than just size separation methods. If the material to be classified could be a mixture of materials of various densities and sizes, the finer part will be richer in the lighter component and the coarser part would be richer in the heavier component.

The process of sedimentation is to settle out all the solids fed and to give a clear overflow. This method is based on the measurement of the particles rate at which it gets settle out from a liquid dispersed. Settling is said to be a process by which particulates gets collected to the bottom of a liquid and form sediment. Settling velocity of a particle also known as fall velocity or terminal velocity is explained as the rate at which the sediment settles in static fluid. It depends on other factors, such as shape of particles, viscosity and density of the fluid. Stokes' Law predicts for dilute suspensions that the settling velocity of small spheres in fluid is either air or water. Stokes' law finds many applications in the natural sciences, and is given by:

$$V = d^2 g (\rho_p - \rho_s)/18\mu$$

where,

V = Settling velocity

ρ = Density (p and f for particle and fluid respectively)

g = Acceleration due to gravity

r = Particle radius

μ = Fluid dynamic viscosity.

A suspension of solids in a liquid is usually water which is placed in a tank and is allowed to stand for a suitable duration of time. Then upper layer is removed which gives a single separation. By arranging the inlet pump the suspension can also be collected as a number of fractions. The pumped suspension will successively contain coarse particles. The main disadvantage of this method is that it is a batch process and it does not give a clear separation of particle sizes. To overcome the above disadvantages, *continuous sedimentation method* may be used. In this method a shallow tank is arranged with inlet and outlet pipe. Particles that are divided into two components—a horizontal component which is due to the flow of the fluid that carries the particles forward and in a vertical component which is due to the gravity that leads the particle to fall down towards the bottom of the tank. It depends on the Stokes' law and due to it; velocity of fall depends on particle size of the particles. Thus, coarse particles get settled closest to the tank and the fine particle near the outlet.

In a few tanks flow is set up in such a manner that only coarse particles gets settle down and the finer particles are carried away by the overflow and gets collected to somewhere else by filtration or sedimentation method.

Elutriation Methods

Principle: In this separation of particles takes place by the movement of a fluid in reverse direction of sedimenting particles.

Construction: It consists of a column having vertical shape and the entry of suspension takes place from the inlet near the bottom and the coarse particles are withdrawn from an outlet located at the base and there is a different outlet at the top to collect fluid and fine particles as depicted in Figs 3.1A and B.

Working: In it separation is obtained into two fractions. It is due to the velocity gradient across the column, particles of different sizes are separated in accordance to the distance from the wall. When more than one fraction is required, a number of

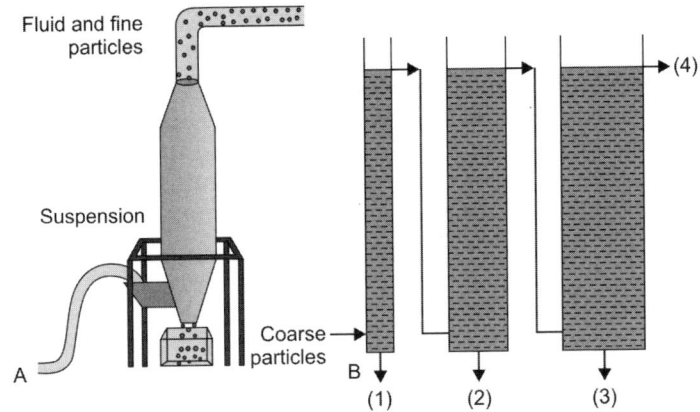

Figs 3.1A and B: A. Elutriation; B. Multi-stage elutriator (1) to (3) is fractions of decreasing particle size

columns of increasing area of cross-section are connected in series. The velocity will decrease in succeeding tubes as the area of cross-section increases, with the same overflow rate and gives a number of fractions.

Uses

- It is used for insoluble solids, e.g. kaolin or chalk that is often subjected to wet grinding followed by elutriation with water
- Also used for finer solids those are separated too slowly in liquids
- It is used for water-soluble substances or even where dry processing is required.

Advantages

- It is a continuous process
- The time require for separation is less than with sedimentation.

Disadvantages: It may be undesirable sometimes or difficult to have a dilute suspension.

SHAKING SCREEN

Principle: In this method of separation different size of particles get separated by passing through a sieve which continuously oscillates in to and fro directions.

Construction: as seen in Fig. 3.2, shaking screen comprises of frame made up of metal having an in-fixed screen at the bottom.

By the help of a removable bolted frame a screen cloth may be engrossed directly or fitted. Metal frame is suspended horizontally or in inclined position by hanger rods to move freely. The complete frame experiences a reciprocating motion as one side of the frame is attached with an ordinary eccentric on a rotating shaft.

Working: The shaking of a screen takes place in a reciprocating motion. The feed is placed on the screen and at first finer particles are screened off whereas leftover particles moves forward and coarse particles are collected from other side.

Advantages

- Low-head room is needed
- Power requirement is much lower.

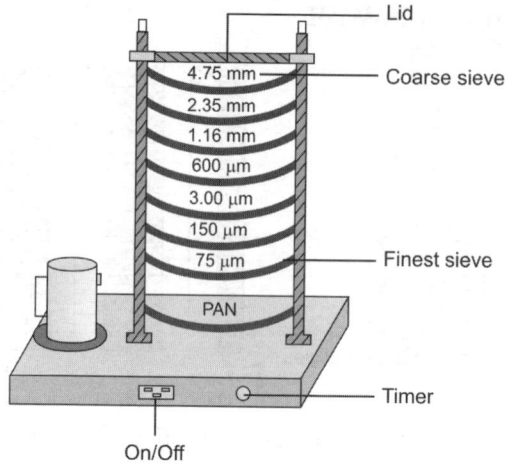

Fig. 3.2: Shaking screen

Disadvantages

- Maintenance cost is high
- Low capacity.

Gyratory Screens

Principle

They are also known as finex. It comprises of a horizontal screen to which a gyratory movement of high intensity and minute amplitude is imparted by eccentric mechanism. On one axis every particle is given a rotary movement and on an another axis at right angles to the first it gives a second rotary movement.

Construction: In it screens are fitted horizontally as shown in Fig. 3.3. The bottom one will have finer opening and the top most has the larger opening. By the help of

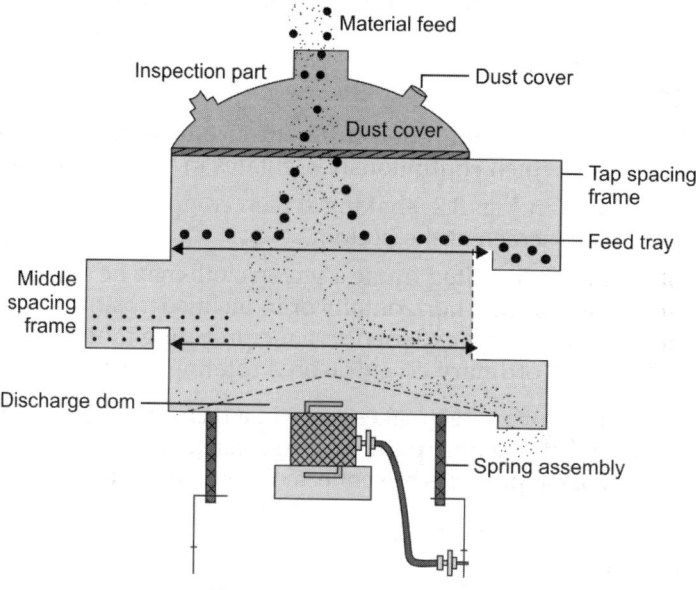

Fig. 3.3: Gyratory screens

eccentric mechanism the complete assembly is given a gyratory motion and on one of the side of the periphery the clearing gates are fitted.

Working: The feed is kept at the middle of the screen and the larger size particles are driven by the gyratory motion towards the periphery of the screen. From the upright side of the sieve it get discharged by a clearing gate. In some devices a metal spiral strip is welded to the screen so that the larger size particles passes dynamically from the middle towards the periphery.

Uses

- In the removal of impurities from wood chips for biomass fuel production
- It is used in the process industry for processing ceramics, pulp and paper mill, paints, sand, starch slurry
- In food industry for screening of refined table salt, papaya cubes, turmeric pigments, clarification of alkaline extracts
- In chemical industry for screening hydrate lime, effluent overflow from hydrocyclone
- It is used in pharmaceuticals industry for manufacturing of formulations and dosage forms.

Advantages

- It has low running cost
- It is considered as ideal for multi-fraction separation
- Has a flexible range of applications
- It provides good efficiency and quality of separation
- Easy to maintained.

Disadvantages

- It requires large amount of floor space
- Relatively hard to operate
- Susceptible to lumps and agglomerates in the feed.

CYCLONE SEPARATOR

Principle: In it separation of the solids from fluids is done by centrifugal force. The solids particle size as well as its density is responsible factors for their separation.

Construction: As seen in Fig. 3.4 cyclone separator consists of a short cylindrical vessel with a base conical in shape and by a tangential inlet upper part is fitted.

The solid outlet is provided at the base and the fluid outlet is at the middle of the top portion that extends inside the separator is used to prevent the direct air short-circuiting of the fluid from the inlet towards the outlet. Such type of arrangement is used to prevent the direct air short-circuiting of the fluid from the inlet towards the outlet.

Working: At fairly high velocity the suspension is introduced tangentially, so that a cyclonic movement takes place within the vessel and the fluid (air) is removed at the top from a central outlet. This cyclonic movement causes the particles to be acted on by centrifugal force, solid being thrown out to the walls, then falling to the conical base and out through it the solids discharge.

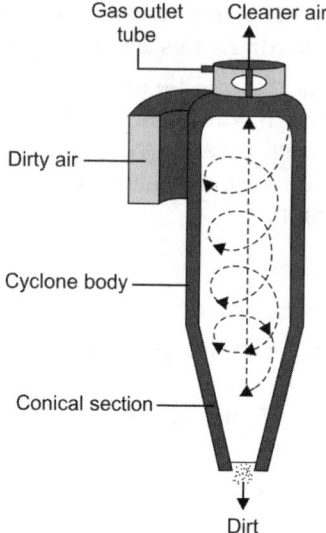

Fig. 3.4: Cyclone separator

Uses

- It is used to separate the solids from gases
- It is also used for separating the heavy or coarse fraction from fine dust
- They act as a part of a group of air pollution control devices known as precleaners
- It is used to separate the solids from liquids.

Advantages

- Inexpensive to install or maintain
- They have no moving parts so maintenance and operating costs is low
- The removed particulate matter is collected when dry so, it is easier to dispose
- Require very little space.

Disadvantages

- The standard models are not able to collect particulate matter that is smaller than 10 micrometers effectively
- The machines are unable to handle sticky or tacky material effectively.

AIR SEPARATOR

Principle: For fine materials only cyclone separator is not sufficient to carry out size separation for these separations a centrifugal force is used with combination of current of air. The coarser particles are thrown by centrifugal force that falls at the bottom while finer particles are carried away by air.

Construction: It consists of a cylindrical vessel having a conical base as shown in Fig. 3.5. At the centre of the vessel a rotating plate is fitted on a shaft placed and a set of fan blades are fitted on the same shaft. At the base of the vessel there are two outlets provided in which one for the coarse particles and the other for finer particles.

Working: The feed (powder) is introduced at the middle of the vessel which falls on the rotating plate. Motor is used to rotate both the fan and the disc. As it is seen

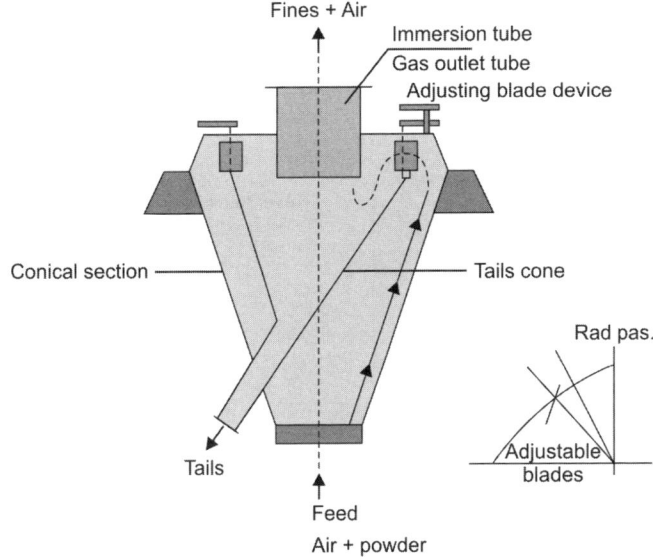

Fines + Air

Immersion tube

Gas outlet tube

Adjusting blade device

Conical section

Tails cone

Rad pas.

Adjustable blades

Tails

Feed

Air + powder

Fig 3.5: Air separator

within the diagram that the a draft (flow) of air in the direction is being produced by the blades of a rotating fan that picks up fine particles and carried them to the space of settling chamber. In it the finer particles are dropped by reducing the air velocity and are removed from the fine particle outlet. Heavy particles are picked up by air stream and are removed at the coarse particle outlet.

Advantages

- Reduction of wear parts
- There is effective separation of bulky waste
- The waste does not interact with the generator of the air flow, avoiding wear and clogging
- Low maintenance cost
- High reliability.

Disadvantages

- Unable to handle sticky or tacky material
- Low efficiency.

BAG FILTER

Principle: Bag filters are also known as bag houses or fabric filters. In it separation of fine particles from the powder is attained in two steps. In first step, the powder is passed on the opposite side of the feed entry through a bag (made from cloth) and to enhance separation suction is applied. In second step, to prevent the adhering of powder from the bag pressure is applied to shake the bags so, that the powder falls off from it, which is then collected from the conical base.

Construction: It comprises of a number of bags as shown in Fig. 3.6 which are made of cotton or wool fabric that is suspended in a metal container. At the top of the metal container, there is a vacuum fan and exhaust through a discharge manifold. At the

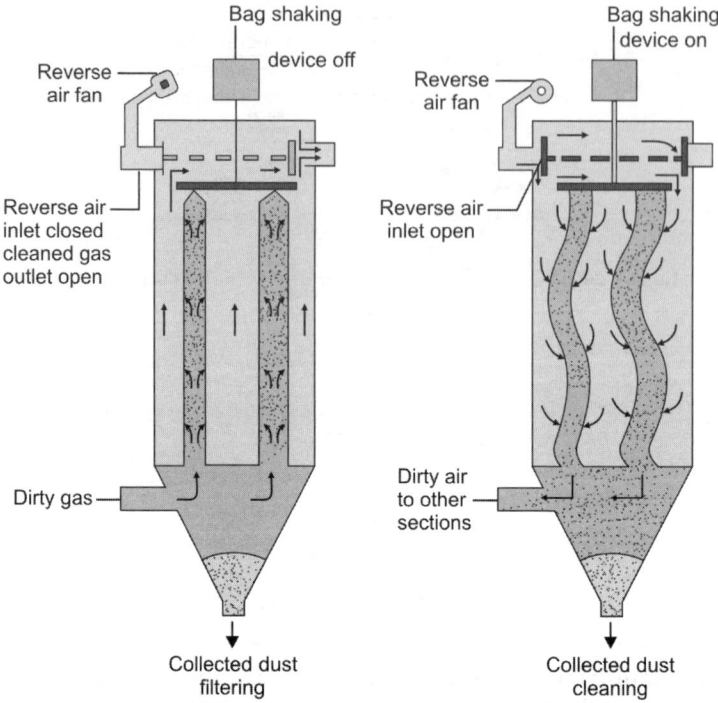

Fig. 3.6: Bag filters

bottom of the filter a hopper is arranged to receive the feed. At the top of the vessel a bell-crank lever arrangement is used to alter the action from filtering to shaking.

Working

a. **Filtering period:** During this period within the vessel, on the vacuum fan a pressure is produced that is lower than the atmospheric pressure. And the gas that is required to be filtered get enters through the hopper and while passing from the bags gets out from the top of the apparatus. And within the bags the particles get retained.

b. **Shaking period:** During this period air enters through the top so the vacuum is broken and firstly the bell-crank lever closes the discharge manifold. At the same time a violent jerking action is given to the bags so, that they can be freed from the dust. At the conical base the fine particles are collected.

Uses

- Bag filter are often used to control the emission of pollutants in power plants, steel mills, pharmaceutical producers, food manufacturers, chemical producers or other industrial companies
- They are also used along with other size separation equipment such as a cyclone separator
- They are use for drying by using the top of fluidized bed dryer to separate the dust particles
- Also helps to clean the air of a room
- A simple version of bag filter is a household vacuum cleaner.

Advantages

- Useful to remove very fine particles
- Easy to clean
- More compact design due to higher filter velocities.

Disadvantages

- Temperature limits the use of fabric filters
- High maintenance costs of bag filters include bag repair and replacement
- They are not size separation equipment
- Limited bag length.

PARTICLE SIZE DISTRIBUTION AND ITS MEASUREMENT

Flow is primary importance when handling a drug powder. When limited amounts of drug are available it can be evaluated by measurements of bulk density and angle of repose. To assess the impact of changes in drug powder properties these are extremely useful derived parameters as new batches become more available. Changes in particle size and shape are generally very apparent; an increase in crystal size or a more uniform shape will lead to a smaller angle of repose and a smaller Carr's index.

Bulk Density

A simple test has been developed to evaluate the flowability of a powder by comparing the poured density and tapped density of a powder and the rate at which it is packed down. A useful empirical guide is given by Carr's compressibility index. This is a simple index that can be determined on small quantities of powder. A similar index has been defined by Hausner. Values less than 1.25 indicate good flow, whereas greater than 1.25 indicates poor flow. Glidant normally improves flow. Carr's index is a one-point determination and does not always reflect the ease or speed with which the powder consolidates. Indeed, some materials have a high index but may consolidate rapidly. Rapid consolidation is essential for uniform filling on tablet machines. An empirical linear relationship exists between the changes in bulk density and the log number of taps.

Angle of Repose

A static heap of powder, with only gravity acting upon it, will tend to form a conical mound. One limitation exists: the angle to the horizontal cannot exceed a certain value, and this is known as the angle of repose (θ). If any particle temporarily lies outside this limiting angle, it will slide down the adjacent surface under the influence of gravity until the gravitational pull is balanced by the friction caused by interparticulate forces. Accordingly, there is an empirical relationship between θ and the ability of the powder to flow. However, the exact value for angle of repose does depend on the method of measurement.

$$\text{Tan } \theta = h/r$$

where,

θ = Angle of repose

h = Height of pile

r = Radius of pile

Carr's Index

The **Carr's index also** known as Carr's compressibility index as it gives an indication of the compressibility of a powder. It is calculated by:

$$C = 100 \; (V_b - V_t/V_b)$$

where,

V_b = Bulk volume of a given mass of powder

V_t = Tapped volume of the same mass of powder

The Carr index is mostly used in pharmaceutics as to measure the flowability of a powder. In a free-flowing powder, the bulk density and tapped density has a close value and therefore, the Carr index would be small. Similarly, in a poor-flowing powder there is greater interparticle interactions, so the difference between the bulk and tapped density observed would be greater and the Carr index would be larger. A Carr index below 15 is considered as good flowability for a powder and greater than 25 is considered as a poor flowability of powder.

Hausner's Ratio

The **Hausner ratio** is defined as a number which is related to the flowability of a powder or of a granular material. It is calculated by:

$$H = \rho T \, / \rho B$$

where,

ρT = Tapped bulk density of a powder

ρB = Freely settled bulk density of a powder

The Hausner ratio value can be change according to the methodology used to determine so, it is not an absolute property of a powder. It is widely used in number of pharmaceutical industries as a measure of the flowability of a powder. A Hausner ratio greater than 1.25 is considered as a poor flowability of a powder.

VERY SHORT QUESTIONS

1. What is size separation? List the objectives and importance.
2. Explain the uses of screen analysis. How it is expressed?
3. What are various grades of coarse powder?
4. Mention the advantages of expressing sieves by a sieve number over the nominal size of aperture.
5. Compare the methods of sieving and classification in terms of their utility.
6. List the method of sieve analysis used for testing powders. Mention relevant advantages.

SHORT QUESTIONS

1. What are standard sieves? List the specifications and standards for sieves as per IP.
2. Differentiate between the following:
   a. Sedimentation and elutriation
   b. Free settling and hindered settling

c. Static and moving liquid methods of elutriation

d. Nominal size of aperture and nominal diameter of the wire

3. **State the term elutriation. What are its advantages and uses?**

4. **Explain particle size distribution and its measurement.**

5. **Detailed the standards fixed by pharmacopoeia for sieves.**

6. **Explain the concept of settling behaviour using water with a suitable example.**

7. **Briefly explain the method of size separation using shaking screens.**

LONG QUESTIONS

1. **Explain the principle, construction, working, uses, advantages and disadvantages of the following:**
   a. Sieve shaker   b. Cyclone separator
   c. Air separator   d. Bag filter
   e. Elutriation tank

2. **Enlist the standards of screens used in pharmaceutical practice with suitable example.**

3. **Describe one industrial method for size separation of powder and its applications.**

4. **Briefly explain the behaviour of slurry setting of thickeners with a suitable diagram.**

5. **Give a detail method using air as a medium for separation.**

6. **Explain the principles of sedimentation of particles using liquid as a medium.**

MULTIPLE CHOICE QUESTIONS

1. **Metal used for making the sieve:**
   a. Zinc   b. Stainless steel
   c. Tin   d. Aluminium

2. **The nature of pharmaceutical powders:**
   a. Monodisperse   b. Polydisperse
   c. Bidisperse   d. None

3. **As per IP-1996, the pharmaceutical powders were classified into ....**
   a. 3   b. 4
   c. 5   d. 6

4. **Most commonly used size separating instrument in laboratory:**
   a. Cyclone separator   b. Sedimentation tank
   c. Sieve shaker   d. All of the above

5. **In sieve shaker, the particles are separated on the basis:**
   a. Particle shape   b. Particle size
   c. Particle diameter   d. Particle density

6. **Modes of motion in size separation:**
   a. Agitation
   b. Brushing
   c. Centrifugal force
   d. All of the above

7. **Sieve number indicates, the number of meshes in:**
   a. 2.54 mm
   b. 25.4 mm
   c. 254 mm
   d. 0.254 mm

8. **As per IP-1996, fine powder should pass through sieve number:**
   a. 10
   b. 22
   c. 44
   d. 85

9. **Screening is a method for separating particles on the basis of:**
   a. Particle size
   b. Particle density
   c. Particle shape
   d. None

10. **Elutriation depends upon the movement of a fluid ....the direction of flow:**
    a. In the same
    b. Against
    c. Perpendicular
    d. None

11. **For coarse sizing, following types of mesh are used:**
    a. Bar screen
    b. Punched plates
    c. Wire sieves
    d. None

12. **Elutriation is a process of:**
    a. Size reduction using mechanical forces
    b. Size separation using a stationary fluid
    c. Size reduction using electrical repelling forces
    d. Size separation using a moving fluid

13. **Equipment in which filtering period and shaking period are alternatively observed:**
    a. Cyclone filter
    b. Bag filter
    c. Edge filter
    d. Air separation

14. **Forces used in cyclone separator for size separation of particles**
    a. Centrifugal forces
    b. Shearing forces
    c. Adhesive forces
    d. Cohesive forces

15. **Disadvantage of sieve shaker method:**
    a. Attrition
    b. Tedious
    c. Capacity limited
    d. Expenses

Heat Transfer |

Md. Abul Kalam and Yasmin Sultana

Heat transfer is a branch of thermal engineering that deals with the generation, use, conversion, and exchange of thermal energy and heat between physical systems. In general, heat transfer is the process which involves the flow of heat under the influence of temperature gradient. Heat energy is not storable, rather it is transferable from hot materials to cold materials. The discussion of heat transfer is not only restricted to the process of heat energy transports but also includes the rate of heat transfer. In the process of evaporation or condensation of a known amount of liquid, the same amount of heat gets transferred but the heat transferring rate in both these processes may differ. A sound knowledge of principles of heat transfer and their applications is helpful for the chemical engineers. Heat transfer is classified into various mechanisms, such as thermal conduction, thermal convection, thermal radiation, and transfer of energy by phase changes.

OBJECTIVES
- To design heat transfer equipment that operates efficiently and economically
- To maintain heat transfer process at industrial scale process
- To investigate the heat flow by conduction (in solid matters), convection (in liquid and gaseous matters) and radiation
- To identify matter classified as conductor and insulator of heat
- To apply the heat flow concept in solving everyday physics problems, such as a vacuum flask and a flat-iron.

APPLICATIONS
The heat is used in pharmaceutical and chemical industries at a large scale, mainly source are steam or electric power. The heat transfer used in various processes such as:
- **Evaporation:** To remove solvent or liquid from extracts, such as vegetables liquid is converted to vapours by heat. Equipment used is known as evaporators, such as shell and tube heat exchanger
- **Distillation:** Heat is supplied to separate different components present in a mixture of liquids to retain desirable products
- **Drying:** Heat is used to remove moisture from the compound, such as tablets or milk products. Equipment used is known as dryers such as tray dryer

- **Crystallisation:** Supersaturation is attained by heating a saturated solution in order to obtain crystals of drugs
- **Sterilization:** Heat is extensively used in sterilization process of various pharmaceuticals, apparatus, containers, etc.
- **Boiling:** A rapid vaporization of a liquid, which occurs when a liquid is heated to its boiling point, it is a temperature at which the vapour pressure of the liquid is equal to the pressure exerted by the surrounding atmosphere on the liquid. Equipment used are boilers in pharmaceutical industry for removal of undesirable dissolved volatile compounds
- **Exsiccation:** Heat is used in process of removal of water of crystallization to obtain pure crystals.

HEAT TRANSFER MECHANISMS

Heat transfer mechanisms are ways by which thermal energy can be transferred between objects and they all rely on the basic principle that kinetic energy or heat required at equilibrium or at *equal energy states.* In the simplest terms, the heat transfer is concerned with two aspects: temperature, and the flow of heat. The temperature shows the amount of thermal energy available, while heat flow corresponds to the movement of thermal energy from one place to another place. The rate at which heat is transferred depends upon the differences in temperature between the bodies, the greater the difference in temperature, the greater the rate of heat transfer.

On microscopic basis, thermal energy of molecules at molecular level, kinetic energy forms the basis of thermal energy of molecules and *vice versa.* When the temperature of a matter increases the kinetic energy of molecules in vibrational modes as well as in linear motion also increases. This phenomenon leads to the transfer of molecular kinetic energy from the region containing higher energy to lower energy, hence the propagation of heat occurs. The common examples of heat transfer are thermal conductivities, fluid viscosities, fluid velocities, specific heats, surface emissivities, material densities. Heat transfer mechanisms can be grouped into three broad categories—**conduction, convection and radiation.**

HEAT TRANSFER BY CONDUCTION

The process of conduction is the transfer of heat from one part of a body to another part of the same body, or between two bodies by means of physical contact, without significant displacement of the particles of the bodies. In other words a region with high molecular kinetic energy passes their thermal energy towards regions of less molecular energy by virtue of direct molecular collisions. A significant portion of the transported thermal energy in metals is carried out by conduction-band electrons.

In it, the following equation can be applied:

$$\text{Rate} = \frac{\text{Driving force}}{\text{Resistance}}$$

The driving force is the temperature difference of heat-transfer path in per unit length, which is also known as the temperature gradient. Instead of resistance to heat flow, its reciprocal used is conductance. The form of general equation is changed to:

$$\text{Rate of heat transfer} = \text{Driving force} \times \text{conductance}$$

That is;

$$\frac{dQ}{dt} = kA\frac{dT}{dx}$$

where,

$\dfrac{dQ}{dt}$ = Rate of heat transfer (the quantity of heat energy transferred per unit time)

A = Area of cross-section of the heat flow path

$\dfrac{dT}{dx}$ = Temperature gradient (rate of change of temperature per unit length of path)

k = Thermal conductivity of the medium

This equation is called the Fourier equation for heat conduction. If the temperature conditions are steady, dQ/dt is constant, which may be called q; **so**

$$q = kA\,\frac{dT}{dx}$$

but dT/dx, the rate change of temperature per unit length of the path, is given by $(T_1-T_2)/x$, where x is the thickness of the slab,

so
$$q = \frac{kA(T_1-T_2)}{x}$$

or
$$q = kA\,\frac{dT}{x}$$

or
$$q = \left(\frac{k}{x}\right)A\Delta T$$

The above equation is the basic equation for simple heat conduction.

FOURIER'S LAW

When there is an existence of temperature gradient within a body, the heat energy will flow from high temperature region to the low temperature region, and the phenomenon is known as conduction heat transfer, which can be described by Fourier's Law (named after the French physicist Joseph Fourier),

$$q = -\kappa\Delta T$$

The above equation is known as Fourier's equation, which determines the heat flux factor 'q' for a given temperature profile 'T' and thermal conductivity 'k'. The minus sign indicates that heat flows down the temperature gradient (ΔT).

HEAT TRANSFER BY CONVECTION

The process of transfer of heat from one point to another point within a medium, or between a fluid and a solid or another fluid, by the movement or mixing of the fluids is known as convection. A local volumetric expansion takes place when heat conducts into a static fluid and as a result of gravity-induced pressure gradients, the expanded fluid becomes buoyant and displaces, thus transports heat by fluidic motion (convection) in addition to conduction, and such kind of heat-induced fluid motion in static fluids is called free convection. If the movement of the fluid is due to differences in density resulting from differences in temperature, then it is known as natural convection. If the motion of the fluid is produced mechanically then the process is known as forced convection (Table 4.1).

Table 4.1: Convective heat transfer coefficients

Convection type	Description	Values of h (W/m²K)
Natural convection	Fluid motion induced by density differences	10 (gas) 100 (liquid)
Forced convection	Fluid motion induced by pressure differences from a fan or pump	100 (gas) 1000 (liquid)

Heating in a jacketed pan without a stirrer is a good example of convection heating. More than one of these modes of heat transfer is needed in most of the cases of transfer of heat energy.

The total rate of heat transfer is expressed in terms of a driving force which is a decrease in temperature and a resistance.

$$\frac{dQ}{dt} = \frac{\text{Driving force}}{\text{Resistance}}$$

$$= \frac{T_1 - T_2}{1} \frac{1}{UA}$$

$$= UA\,(T_1 - T_2)$$

where,

$\dfrac{dQ}{dt}$ = Rate of heat transfer (as in Btu/hr) in the direction from point 1 to 2

t = Time (h)

T_1 and T_2 = Temperatures at points 1 and 2 respectively (°F)

U = Average overall coefficient of heat transfer (as in Btu/hr ft²°F)

A = Area of surface through which heat is transferred, or cross-sectional area of material through which heat is being conducted (as in sq ft.)

The flow of heat or electrical energy may be considered as controlled by a driving force and a resistance. The driving force for electrical energy is the difference in potential called voltage, and for heat energy the driving force is the difference in temperature. The rate of flow of electricity through several resistances in series is obtained by dividing the voltage by the sum of the resistances;

$$I = \frac{E}{R}$$

where,

I = Rate of electrical flow

E = Driving force, voltage

R = Resistance

Likewise, the rate of flow of heat for a series of resistances is expressed by the equation:

$$\frac{dQ}{dt} = \frac{T_1 - T_2}{R_{1-2} + R_{1-3} + R_{1-4}}$$

$$= \frac{T_1 - T_2}{(K_{1-2})^{-1} + (K_{2-3})^{-1} + (K_{3-4})^{-1}}$$

where,

R = Resistance

K = Conductance

The proper overall coefficient U is determined by the expression,

$$\frac{1}{UA}=(K_{1-2})^{-1}+(K_{2-3})^{-1}+(K_{3-4})^{-1}$$

or the total resistance is equal to the sum of the individual resistances for series law.

HEAT TRANSFER BY RADIATION

Radiation is the transfer of heat by the absorption of radiant energy. The vibrations in the molecules generate electromagnetic radiation, the amount of which is related to the temperature of the object. The radiation transmits energy through space and vacuum, and when it impacts on other molecules some of this radiation (energy) is absorbed by the receiving molecules. Electromagnetic waves emanate from all bodies in all directions at all temperatures. The most important property of electromagnetic waves is that they convey energy. When the waves impinge on a body, some parts are reflected, some parts are transmitted, and some parts are absorbed. The absorbed waves may be converted into high-grade forms of energy as in photochemical changes, but they are more commonly converted into heat. Light is also due to similar radiant energy but of shorter wavelength or higher frequency. Electromagnetic waves emitted by the sun travel through space in straight lines to furnish both heat and light to the earth.

STEFAN-BOLTZMANN LAW

All materials radiate thermal energy in such amounts that is known by their temperature, in which the energy is carried by photons of light in the infrared and visible spectrum of the electromagnetic radiation. The radiative flux between objects is in equilibrium when temperatures are uniform and there is exchange of any net thermal energy. The balance is disturbed when temperatures are not uniform throughout, and thermal energy is transported from planes of higher to planes of lower temperature.

The intensity of radiation emitted from a black body (those bodies which absorb all the incident energy) depends solely upon the fourth power of the absolute temperature. This relationship is known as the Stefan-Boltzman law and this is the basic formula of radiant heat transfer. The intensity of radiation from a nonblack body depends upon the emissivity of that body as well as upon the fourth power of its absolute temperature. The energy emitted from a unit area of a body to the whole hemisphere which it sees is;

$$E=\frac{q}{A}=e\sigma T^4$$

where,

e = Emissivity (unity for a black body)

σ = Stefan-Boltzman constant [1730×10^{-12} in Btu/(sq ft) (hr) (degree Rankine)^4]

T = Absolute temperature of the body

This law gives the radiation emitted by a black body (perfect radiator which gives the maximum quantity of emitted radiation possible at its particular temperature). The above equation can be rewritten as:

$$q = eA\sigma T^4$$

where, e is called emissivity of the particular body and is a number between 0 and 1. This equation is obeyed by grey bodies.

A black body emits a continuous series of wavelengths with the maximum intensity at wavelengths from 1 to 5 micrometers, depending upon the temperature. The *emissivity 'e'* is the ratio of energy which a body emits relative to the energy emitted by a perfect radiator (black body) of the same area and at the same temperature. The *absorptivity 'a'* is the ratio of the energy absorbed by a body to the energy absorbed by a black body of the same area under the same condition. The *absorptivity 'a'* of a surface depends upon the nature of the surface and upon the distribution of the wavelengths in the incident radiation. The *emissive power 'E'* of the surface is the total energy emitted, per unit area, unit time. The *intensity 'i'* of radiation is the amount of energy emitted per unit area, unit time, unit solid angle.

KIRCHHOFF'S LAW

Kirchhoff's law of heat transfer by radiation states that for a particular surface area for thermal equilibrium the monochromatic absorptivity (α_λ) is equal to the monochromatic emissivity (ε_λ).

During the years 1860–1862, Kirchhoff stated a theoretical object (black body), a body that can absorb 100% radiation falling on its surface at all wavelengths and this black body could emit a continuous spectrum of radiation in such a way that the emission intensity at any given wavelength will depend only on the absolute temperature and the wavelength of the black body. More precisely, this law can be elaborated as, e.g. a cold metal cube was put near a hot metal similar cube, the hot cube will emit a lot of heat but absorb very little amount of heat from the cold cube. After sometimes, both the cubes will reach to the equal temperature, and at that instance, the radiation form hot cube will be equal to cold cube and at the same moment the output and input radiation are equal, therefore α_λ will be equal to ε_λ.

HEAT INTERCHANGERS

Heat interchangers are equipment used for transferring heat from one gas to a different or from one liquid to a different by a metal wall. They are additionally called heat transfer equipment. In heat interchangers, the heating medium could be a hot liquid and the liquid to be heated is the cold liquid. During this case, the film coefficients each outside and within are measure nearly of same magnitude. The worth of overall heat transfer constant, U, are close to that of the smaller of the 2 film coefficients. Hence, heat transfer is not efficient. The film coefficients are also increased by increasing the velocity of flow. From the purpose of construction, it is tough to extend the velocity of the fluid from outside the tubes. However, surface area of contact may be raised by introducing baffles within the construction and also enhances the constant. So, the rate of heat transfer is increased. These principles help to illustrate different heat interchangers.

Baffles: It consists of circular discs of flat solid with one facet cut away and are perforated to receive tubes. To reduce leak, the clearance between baffles, shell and tubes ought to be little. They are supported by one or more guide rods, which are fixed by set-screws between the tubes.

Working: They are placed outside the tubes and help to increase the rate of liquid outside the tubes. It makes the liquid flow at right angles to the tubes, that creates a lot of turbulence and this helps in minimising the resistance to heat transfer outside the tubes. So, it is considered as an important part in heat transfer. It is more justified in construction of liquid to liquid heat interchanger.

LIQUID TO LIQUID HEAT INTERCHANGER

All heat transfer equipment nearly has same construction and working with a few modifications.

Construction: It has tube sheets, spacer rods, baffles assembled first and then tubes are installed as illustrated in Fig. 4.1, the essential part is baffles. Appopriate size of tube sheets are choosen for fabrication. One or more guide rods are fixed by means of set-screws. Baffles consist of circular discs of sheet metal with one side cut away. And are then placed at appropriate place by making use of guide rods and are arranged with appropriate spacing using short sections of the same tubing. The ends of tubes are expanded into the tube sheets.

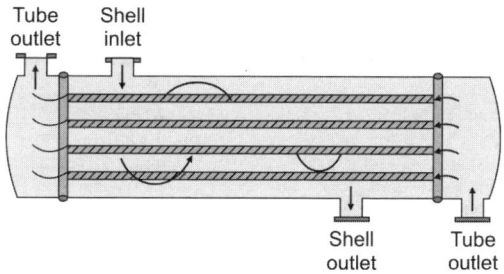

Fig. 4.1: Liquid to liquid heat interchanger

The whole assembly is enclosed in a shell having provision for introducing the heating medium or hot fluid. At top right side there is outlet for the fluid. On either side of the tubes there are 2 distribution chambers. Left side contains an inlet for fluid to be heated while at the centre of the right side of the distribution chamber, the outlet for a hot fluid (i.e. heated) is provided.

Working: From the left side top of the shell, a hot fluid (i.e. heated medium) is pumped up. The fluid flows moves down directly to the bottom flowing from outside the tubes. Then, it changes the direction once more. This method is sustained until it leaves the heater. Baffles increase the rate of transfer of liquid outside the tubes and also enable the fluid to flow more or less at right angles to the tube, that creates a lot of turbulence. These facilitate in reducing the resistance to heat transfer outside the tubes. Baffles lengthen the path and reduce the cross-section of path of the cold fluid. The baffles get heated and provide a large surface area for transfer of heat. Throughout the flow, the tubes conjointly get heated. As a result, the film constant within the tube conjointly will increase.

Through the inlet involved on left side distribution chamber, liquid to be heated is pumped. The liquid passes through the tubes and gets heated and have flow of liquid as a single pass. The heated liquid is collected from the right side of the distribution chamber.

Advantages

Heat transfer is rapid as liquid passes at high velocities outside tube.

DOUBLE PIPE HEAT INTERCHANGER

In a liquid to liquid heat interchanger, the fluid to be heated is passed only once through the tubes before it gets discharged, i.e. single pass. The heat transfer in this case is not efficient. When a few tubes per pass is desirable, double pipe heat interchanger is employed.

Construction: It consists of two pipes that are inserted in one other. The inner pipe/tube is used for the pumping of cold liquid to be heated while outer pipe of the hot liquid acts as a jacket for the circulation. All sections of jacket are interconnected (Fig. 4.2).

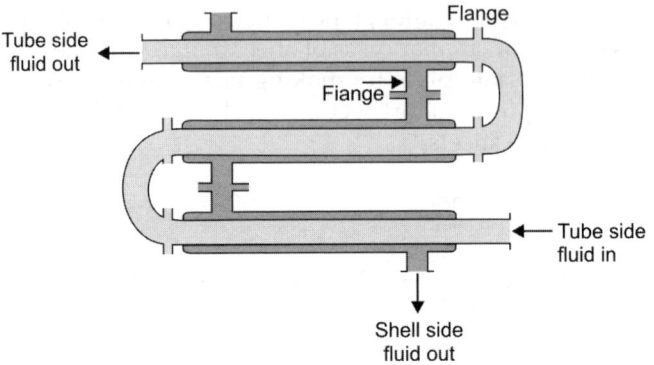

Fig. 4.2: Double pipe heat interchanger

Mainly, there are a few number of pipe sections, having the less length of the pipe. They are made up of glass tube, standard iron pipe and graphite. Standard metal pipes are always assembled with standard return bends. A proper number of such pipes are stacked vertically and are connected in parallel. On its outer surface these pipes might have longitudinal fins.

Working: The hot liquid is pumped-up into the jacketed section. The hot fluid is circulated through the annulate areas between them and carried from one section to other and leaves the jacket finally. In this method the pipes get heated, whereas the hot fluid looses its temperature.

The liquid to be heated is pumped up through the inlet provided at right side of equipment. The liquid gets heated and flows through the bent tubes inside the next section of the pipe and further gets heated. An equivalent liquid continues to flow and eventually leaves the interchanger through the exit outlet on right side of the chamber.

Advantage: It is useful when not more than 0.9 to 1.4 m² of surface is required.

HEAT EXCHANGERS

The nomenclature, heat transfer refers to any or all styles of instrumentation within which transfer of heat is performed from one medium to a different medium. A domestic radiator, wherever hot water provides up its heat to the close air, could be an ideal of this device. Also, a boiler wherever combustion gases quit their heat to water so as to attain evaporation is also represented. A boiler can also be considered as an example for heat exchanger. In boiler the heat generation occurs by combustion of coal which generates heat required to raise the temperature of water in the tubes and produce steam. Due to the principle followed, it is also known as fire tube heat exchanger. Whereas in case of heat exchangers, the steam itself act as a heating material responsible for heating the tube or plate surface for further application. A shell and tube heat exchanger is an example of non-storage calorifier as it is used as a space heater. A storage calorifier differs from non-storage calorifier with respect to its construction and the presence of its heating coil inside water storage vessel. Figure 4.3

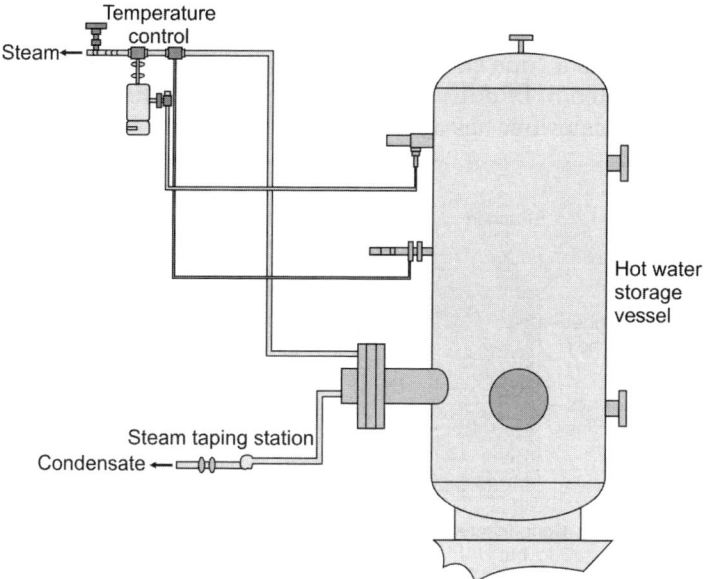

Fig. 4.3: An outline of a storage calorifier installation

explains the construction of a storage calorifier and the thermal energy produced is expressed in terms of kilowatt (kW). Although the heat exchangers are generally huge in sizes in order to provide maximum output but still plate heat exchangers are available in various standard sizes by modifying the manner they are welded together and the number of plates arranged. If the number of plates are increased or decreased, it has a direct effect on the heat transfer as it will affect the surface area. Most of the heat exchangers are kept oversize just to prevent the reduction in pressure for the fluid.

On contrary, the representative examples of flow type applications are shell and tube heat exchangers as well as plate heat exchangers.

Tubular Heat Exchangers

The shell and tube heat exchanger is taken into account because the most typical technique of providing indirect heat exchange within the processes of industrial applications. The above mentioned heat exchangers are mainly made up of circular tubes, however based on the requirement or application twisted, round, flat, rectangular or elliptical tubes have also been designed. Furthermore, alteration in tube length, diameter and arrangement helps in varying the core geometry and ultimately provides significant flexibility to the exchanger. Design of tubular heat exchanger is of great importance when the relative pressure of fluid is higher than atmospheric pressure and when pressure difference of two fluids are high. The tubular heat exchangers are mainly used for the heat transfer from a liquid to another liquid and from a liquid phase to a modified phase (such as condensate or vapor). They have also been utilized for the heat transfer from a gas to another gas and from a gas to a liquid particularly when the working pressure or temperature is great degree high and fouling is an extreme issue on at least one side of liquid. Some of the examples of tubular heat exchangers are spiral tube exchanger, shell and tube exchanger and double-pipe exchanger. Except for exchangers having fins outside/inside tubes they are all known to be prime surface exchangers.

Steam Heated Non-storage Calorifiers

They are also known as a "one shell pass two tube pass" kind of shell and tube heat exchanger and consisted of bundles of U-tubes fitted into a fixed tube sheet. A steam to water non-storage calorifier has a common design like as shown in Fig. 4.4

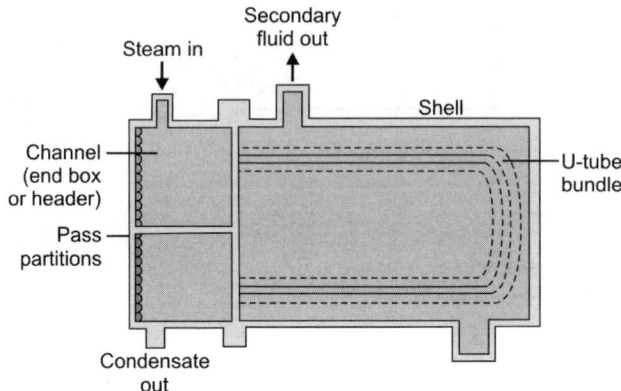

Fig. 4.4: Schematic diagram of a shell and tube heat exchanger

It is known as "one shell pass" when the inlet and outlet for tube side fluid are not present at the same side of instruments, the secondary fluid travels the shell side fluid only once and hence known as "one tube pass". Furthermore, the instrument is called as "two tube passes" when both inlet and outlet for tube side fluid are present at the same side of instruments. On the other hand, when there is no internal baffle present in the shell side it is known as "one shell pass" whereas one internal baffle present in the shell side makes the instrument "two shell pass" because in this case primary fluid passes the shell twice. Usually a partition plate is provided to divide the header of exchanger. It helps in diverting the fluid down the U-tube bundles. This arrangement is simple and less expensive as just a single tube sheet is needed, yet have constrained utilize. Extremely hard to clean so just clean liquids are utilized. A shell and tube exchanger is depicted in Fig. 4.4 may be used as an internal floating head and is more adaptable than the fixed head U-tube exchangers. For the applications of higher temperature differences between the steam and the secondary fluid they show better performance. They are easily cleaned as the tube bundle can be safely removed. Generally to increase the length of the flow path the tube-side fluid is directed to flow through a number of passes.

Mainly exchangers are made of 1–16 tube passes, and the number of passes is being chosen according to the designed tube-side velocity. A number of partition plates are used for dividing up the header in the tubes that are arranged into the number of passes needed. In two shell passes, longitudinal baffles are used to direct the flow of fluids through the shell side. This arrangement is important for insufficient fluid flow volume and when the difference in temperature not enough for a single pass. Furthermore, when the pressure of fluid is more crucial than heat transfer rate, in that case split flow or divided flow is more helpful. In order to decrease the shell-side pressure drop. Reboiler is a one type of shell and tube heat exchanger in which steam might be used to evaporate a liquid. It is mostly used in the petroleum industry to evaporate from the distillation column, a fraction of the bottom product. They are placed horizontally in which vaporisation takes place in the shell and condensation in the tubes (Fig. 4.5).

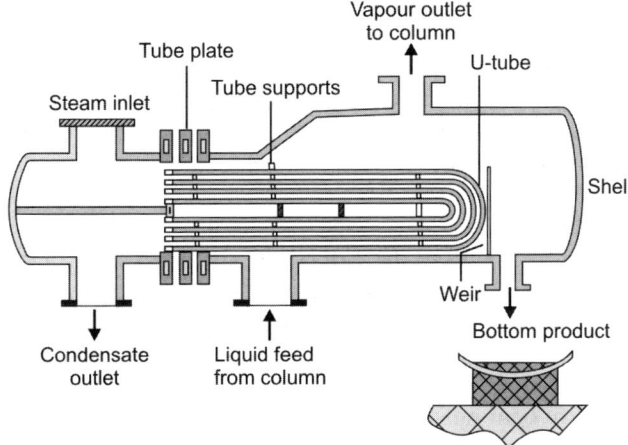

Fig. 4.5: A kettle reboiler

The secondary fluid is pumped forcefully through the exchanger in a forced circulation reboilers and in thermosyphon reboilers natural circulation is maintained by differences in density of different fluids. In the kettle reboilers, the tubes are immersed in a pool of liquid and there is no circulation of the secondary fluid. Characteristic heat transfer coefficients for some shell and tube heat exchangers can be presented as in Table 4.2.

Corrugated Tube Heat Exchangers

It is a single passage fixed plate heat exchanger with a welded shell, and rectilinear corrugated tubes appropriate for having low viscosity fluids. They promote turbulent in operation conditions which increases heat transfer and reduce in a similar manner as the plate heat exchangers does. Similarly to the conventional shell and tube heat exchangers, these units are typically installed horizontally, however within the corrugated tube heat exchanger the steam is usually be on the shell side.

Spiral Heat Exchangers

The construction of spiral heat exchanger provides an extra edge over other heat exchangers due to its large surface area. This heat exchanger is fabricated by folding and welding two long metallic plates in such a way that they make two separate but

Table 4.2: Characteristic heat transfer coefficients for some shell and tube heat exchangers

Secondary fluids	Heat transfer coefficients U $(W/m^2 °C)$
Water	1500–4000
Organic solvents	500–1000
Light oils	300–900
Heavy oils	60–450
Gases	30–300
Aqueous solutions (vaporizing)	1000–1500
Light organics (vaporizing)	900–1200
Heavy organics (vaporizing)	600–900

concentric spiral channels. No intermixing of fluids is assured by welding the edges of plates and according to the requirement, gap between plates and width of channel plate are optimized. Both the fluids flowing inside the separated spiral channels experience very high turbulence which also enhances the effectiveness of heat transfer. The high shear rate based self-cleaning facility makes it suitable for heavy slurries and fouling fluids that are very heavy.

Plate Heat Exchangers

They are typically design of thin plates (all prime surfaces). They are either smooth or have some type of corrugation, and that they are either flat or wound in an **associate degree** exchange. Generally, these exchangers cannot accommodate pressure and temperature differences or very high pressures temperatures. It is comprised of a progression of thin corrugated or wrinkled metal plates arranged in a manner that they automatically form channels. The cold and hot liquid are allowed to flow parallel to each other in the subsequent plates. As the plates are conductive in nature the heat transfer takes place from the hot liquid to the cold liquid (Fig. 4.6).

Plate heat exchangers (PHEs) can be classified as gasketed, welded (one or both fluid passages), or brazed, depending on the leak tightness required. Other plate-type exchangers are spiral plate, lamella, and plate coil exchangers.

The corrugated/furrowed pattern of ridges will increase the rigidity of the plates and offers bigger support against the differential pressures. This kind of arrangement creates turbulent flow within the channels, improves heat transfer efficiency, which successively builds. This sort of arrangement generates turbulent stream inside the channels and enhances the effectiveness of heat exchange. Due to this compact structure, plate heat exchanger is more efficient than a tube compose heat exchanger and standard shell. The reinforcement of turbulent stream additionally wipes out the nearness of stagnant zones and in this manner decreases dirt and any harm. The metal plates are at times covered on the primary side, in order to empower the dropwise condensation of steam. This helps in providing the sub-cooling of condensate as well as condensing inside the single unit loss of flash steam to the atmosphere through the receiver vent is also reduced when the condensate is drained to an atmospheric receiver by reducing the condensate temperature. And this could eliminate the requirement of a separate sub-cooler or flash steam recovery system.

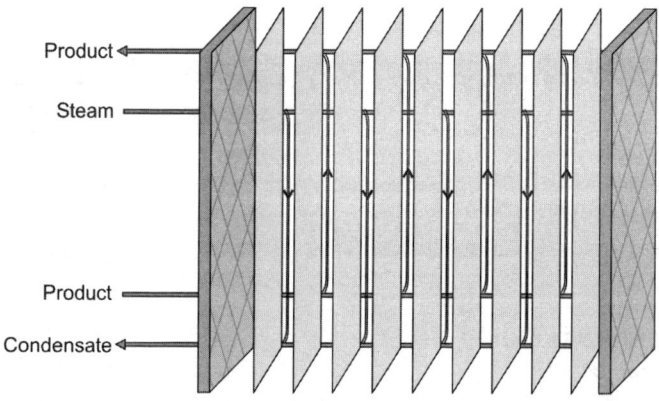

Fig. 4.6: Schematic diagram of a plate heat exchanger

Gasketed Plate Heat Exchangers (Plate and Frame Heat Exchangers)

In this exchanger the plates are clamped along in a frame, every plate is sealed around the edge with the thin gaskets (these gaskets are generally made of synthetic polymers). To compress the plate pack between the frame plate and therefore, the pressure plate tightening bolts are fitted and such type of design allows simple *disassembling* of the units for cleaning. Also it allows the modification in the units' capacity by easily adding or removal of the plates. The gaskets are used because they provide a degree of flexibility to the plate packing which offer resistance to thermal fatigue and for sudden changes in the pressure. This is the reason for gasketed plate heat exchanger to become an ideal choice as a steam heater for instant supply of hot water, wherever the plates are exposed to a certain amount of thermal cycling.

Brazed Plate Heat Exchangers

In it all the plates are brazed together using a hard solder (mostly copper or nickel) in a vacuum furnace. The brazed plate heat exchanger is an advancement of the gasketed plate heat exchanger, and it was developed with an intention to provide more resistance to higher pressures and temperatures at cost-effective price.

But as the gasketed unit can be dismantled, the brazed plate heat exchanger cannot be disassembled for cleaning and other purposes. When cleaning is needed then it must be cleaned chemically or back-flushed. Moreover oversizing is very common in these units as they are available in a standard range of sizes.

They are primarily used for applications where variations in temperature are too slow, such as in case of space heating. They can be used successfully with secondary fluids where there is gradual expansion of fluid occurs, e.g. thermal oil.

Welded Plate Heat Exchangers

In it the plate packing is held tightly together by welded seems between the plates. But in this laser welding techniques are used that allows the plate pack to be more flexible as compared to a brazed plate pack and thus, the welded unit is more resistant to pressure pulsation and thermal cycling. Its operation at higher temperature and pressure limits of the welded unit mean that these normally have a higher specification, and are much more suitable for heavy duty processes in industrial applications. They are generally used where a higher pressure and or higher temperature performance is needed, or when the viscous media are to be heated, e.g. oil and other hydrocarbons.

VERY SHORT QUESTIONS

1. **Explain types of condensation for saturated vapour free from non-condensable gases.**

2. **Differentiate between:**
   a. Black body and grey body
   b. Heat interchanger and heat exchanger
   c. Dry saturated steam and superheated steam

3. **Define entrainment and how it is prevented?**

4. **Describe the types of heat transfer mechanism.**

5. **List the characteristics of heat transfer by radiation.**

6. **What is overall heat transfer coefficient?**

SHORT QUESTIONS

1. What is heat transfer? State its objectives and applications.

2. Explain the following:
   a. Fourier's law
   b. Stefan Boltzaman's law
   c. Kirchoff's law

3. Describe heat exchangers with suitable example and its advantages.

4. Explain heat transfer mechanism with suitable equations.

5. Write a note on tubular heat exchangers.

6. Classify heat interchangers with suitable example.

LONG QUESTIONS

1. Describe finned tube heat exchanger in detail with its specific advantages?

2. Derive an equation for heat transfer through a circular pipe with a suitable law?

3. Explain construction and working of following:
   a. Double pipe heat interchanger   b. Shell and tube heat exchanger
   c. Steam heated non storage calorifiers   d. Liquid to liquid heat interchanger
   e. Plate heat exchanger

4. Elaborate plate heat exchangers.

5. Explain heat transfer by conduction in detail.

MULTIPLE CHOICE QUESTIONS

1. Which of the following are compact heat exchangers?
   a. Double-pipe exchanger   b. Automobile radiator
   c. Plate exchanger   d. Sterling engine regenerator

2. Which of the following has high thermal conductivity?
   a. Stainless steel   b. Steel
   c. Glass   d. Copper

3. Baffles are used primarily to:
   a. Increase cross-section of path   b. Decrease turbulence
   c. Increase path travel   d. None

4. A finned double-pipe exchanger has fins on the outside of the inner tube(s) for the following reasons:
   a. The tube outside heat transfer coefficient is high
   b. The tube inside heat transfer coefficient is more than double for tube outside with longitudinal flow
   c. Fouling is expected on the tube side
   d. None

5. **Which one of the following is not a function fulfilled by transverse plate baffles in a shell-and-tube exchanger?**
   a. To provide counter flow operation
   b. To support the tubes
   c. To direct the fluid approximately at right angles to the tubes
   d. To increase the turbulence and mixing in the shell fluid
   e. To minimize tube-to-tube temperature differences and thermal stresses

6. **Which one is responsible for heat transfer by natural convection:**
   a. Agitation
   b. Surface area
   c. Density of vapour
   d. Material of construction

7. **Which of the following properties of plate heat exchangers, due to their specific construction features, make them particularly suited for the food processing industry?**
   a. Close temperature control
   b. Easy disassembly for cleaning
   c. Low probability of one fluid to other fluid contamination
   d. High corrosion resistance

8. **Which of the following equipment uses heat transfer by radiation?**
   a. Incubator
   b. Hot air oven
   c. Microwave oven
   d. Refrigerator

9. **Fourier's law is used to:**
   a. Conduction
   b. Radiation
   c. Convection
   d. None

10. **Mechanism used in the hot air oven through a fan:**
    a. Conduction and forced convection
    b. Conduction and natural convection
    c. Conduction, radiation and forced convection
    d. Radiation and forced convection

11. **A medium most effective for thermal radiation:**
    a. Air
    b. Water
    c. Vacuum
    d. Insulated with cotton

12. **A heat interchanger highly efficient is:**
    a. Double pipe heater
    b. Multi pass heater
    c. Two pass floating head heater
    d. Tubular heater

13. **In SI unit 1 atm is equivalent to:**
    a. 101
    b. 100
    c. 1
    d. 1001

14. **Thermal conductivity and resistance of metals are related in the following proportionality:**
    a. Logarithmically
    b. Exponentially
    c. Inversely
    d. Directly

15. **Which of the following types of steam is used as a heating medium**
    a. Exhaust steam
    b. Wet steam
    c. Superheated steam
    d. Saturated steam.

16. **Which of the following is not a property of heat waves?**
    a. Ability to travel in a straight line
    b. Ability to be reflected in a mirror
    c. Ability to pass through air
    d. Ability to pass through a vacuum

17. **................. are not considered as opaque surfaces in radiation:**
    a. Gases
    b. Liquids
    c. Solids
    d. None

18. **Black surfaces are good for .... heat transfer.**
    a. Conduction
    b. Radiation
    c. Both a and b
    d. Convection

19. **Fourier's law explains heat transfer due to:**
    a. Convection
    b. Conduction
    c. Radiation
    d. Both a and b

20. **Convective heat transfer normally occurs in:**
    a. Gases
    b. Liquids
    c. Fluids
    d. All above

21. **Kirchhoff's law is used in .... radiation.**
    a. Alpha
    b. Total
    c. Gamma
    d. All above

22. **The units for the log mean temperature difference are:**
    a. °C
    b. 1/°C
    c. Dimensionless
    d. °F

23. **Thermal conductivity of a given liquid dependent on:**
    a. Viscosity
    b. Temperature
    c. Pressure
    d. Height

24. **The evaporator economy is dependent on the:**
    a. Mass transfer rate
    b. Heat transfer rate
    c. Energy balance considerations
    d. None

MATHEMATICAL PROBLEMS ON HEAT TRANSFER

Problem 1

A 22 feet uninsulated steam line crosses a room. The outer diameter of the steam line is 18 inches and the outer surface temperature is 280°F. The convective heat transfer coefficient for the air is 18 Btu/h.ft^{-2}.°F. What will be the rate of heat transfer from the pipe into the room if the room temperature was 72°F.

Solution:

The rate heat transfer, dQ/dt from the pipe into the room can be calculated as,

$$\frac{dQ}{dt} = UA(T_1 - T_2)$$

$$\frac{dQ}{dt} = U \times 2\pi r L(T_1 - T_2)$$

$$\frac{dQ}{dt} = 18 \text{ Btu/h.ft}^{-2} \times 2(3.14)(0.75\text{ft})(22\text{ft})(280 - 72°F)$$

$$\frac{dQ}{dt} = 3.88 \times 10^5 \text{ Btu/h}$$

Problem 2

Example

If the surface temperature of the sun is 5800 K and if we assume that the sun can be regarded as a black body the radiation energy per unit time can be expressed by the Stefan-Boltzmann equation, where σ is the Stefan-Boltzmann constant (σ = 5.6703 × 10⁻⁸ W/m²K⁴)

$$q = \sigma T^4 A$$

$$q = (5.6703 \times 10^{-8})(5800)^4$$

$$q = 6.42 \times 10^{-7} \text{ W/m}^2$$

Problem 3

A long pipe of 0.6 m outside diameter is buried in earth with axis at a depth of 1.8 m. The surface temperature of pipe and earth are 950 and 250°C respectively. Calculate the heat loss from the pipe per unit length. The conductivity of earth is 0.51 W/mK, find heat loss from the pipe (Q/L)

Solution:

Given that,

$$r = \frac{0.6}{2} = 0.3\,m$$

$$L = 1 \text{ m}, D = 1.8 \text{ m}$$

$$T_p = 95°C, T_e = 25°C$$

$$k = 0.51 \text{ W/mK}$$

We know that heat loss from the pipe (Q/L) can be expressed as,

$\frac{Q}{L} = k.S(T_p - T_e)$, where S is the conduction shape factor

hence,

$$S = \frac{2\pi L}{\ln \dfrac{2D}{r}}$$

$$S = \frac{2\pi \times 1}{\ln \dfrac{2 \times 1.8}{0.3}}$$

$$S = 2.528 \text{ m}$$

now,

$$\frac{Q}{L} = 0.51 \times 2.528(95 - 25)$$

so,

$$\frac{Q}{L} = 90.25 \text{ W/m}$$

Problem 4

What will be the frictional heat Q, if a cylinder of 1 mm diameter loaded with 100 g weight is sliding over a mild steel surface with a velocity of 100 cms^{-1}, when the measured value of the kinetic friction is 0.23.

Solution:

The amount of frictional heat Q is given by,

$$Q = \mu \frac{Wgv}{j}$$

$$Q = \frac{0.23 \times 100 \times 981}{4.2 \times 10^7} \text{ Calorie } S^{-1}$$

$$Q = 5.37 \times 10{-}2 \text{ Calorie } S^{-1}$$

Evaporation

Yasmin Sultana and Md. Aqil

The operation of evaporation is usually defined as the concentration of solution by evaporation in vapor heated equipment. Evaporators depend entirely upon heat transfer for their operation.

Scaling is the term normally used in reference to deposition of a solid whose solubility decreases with increasing temperature on the heating surface from the hotter liquor adjacent to the heating surface.

Salting is a rapid buildup of a normally soluble material on the heating surface in the zone of vaporization. It is aggravated by small fluctuations in the operating conditions and by any condition that will encourage crystal nucleation, rather than the deposition of materials on previously formed crystals.

EVAPORATION AND OTHER HEAT PROCESS

The residue in evaporation process is a concentrated liquid, in drying the residue is a solid. In evaporation, evaporating liquid is only one component but, in *distillation*, *e*vaporating liquid is a combination of two or more components. The product of evaporation is concentrated liquid but in crystallization, the product is solid crystals.

OBJECTIVES

- To concentrate solution consisting of non volatile solute and volatile solvent.
- To reduce the volume of the product without loss of major components.
- To effectively and efficiently remove large amounts of moisture.
- To remove moisture content from thermolabile drugs without affecting its quality.

APPLICATIONS

Manufacture of bulk drugs: Evaporation process is used for the production of bulk drugs.

Manufacture of biological products: Evaporation is used in the preparation of biological products, such as insulin, biochemical products (e.g. penicillin), enzymes, hormones, antibiotics and plant products. Blood products, such as blood plasma and serum are also prepared by evaporation.

Preparation of de-mineralized water: Water containing minerals is subjected to evaporation to get demineralized water after condensation. The process is generally called distillation.

FACTORS INFLUENCING EVAPORATION

The rate of evaporation depends on several factors; the relationship may be expressed mathematically as:

$$M = \frac{KS}{P}\,(b-b^1)$$

where

M = Mass of vapor formed per unit time (rate), m³/s
S = Surface area of the liquid exposed, m²
P = Atmospheric pressure, kPa
b = Maximum vapour pressure at the temperature of air, kPa
b^1 = Pressure due to the vapour of the liquid, actually present in the air, kPa
K = Constant, m/s

In general mass transfer also depends on the temperature.

Temperature

The higher the temperature, the greater is the maximum vapour pressure at the temperature of air (b) and hence greater will be the evaporation.

At a particular temperature, some molecules possess higher kinetic energy than average, while others have lower than average kinetic energy. Fast moving molecules escape from the surface of the liquid into vapour, but slow moving ones remain behind. When temperature of the liquid is increased, more molecules acquire sufficient kinetic energy and escape from the surface of liquid to vapour state. This occurs below the boiling point of the liquid.

Below boiling point, vapour is formed from the surface only. At boiling point, vapour is formed throughout the body of the liquid as well as from surface. The vapour pressure of a liquid is lowered when a substance is dissolved in it and as a result of it boiling point of the liquid increases.

Generally, glycosides and alkaloids decompose at high temperature. Hormones, enzymes and antibiotics are even more heat-sensitive. During evaporation, these products require special techniques to prevent decomposition. For example, malt extract is prepared by evaporation under reduced pressure to avoid loss of enzymes. Antibiotics are concentrated by freeze-drying.

Vapour Pressure

Rate of evaporation is directly proportional to the vapour pressure of the liquid. The lower the atmospheric pressure (p) in the above equation the greater the evaporation. Lower the external pressure, the lower the boiling point of the liquid and hence greater will be the rate of evaporation. This condition is achieved by applying vacuum.

The rate of evaporation is also affected by the nature of liquid. Liquids with low boiling points evaporate quickly because of high vapour pressure at lower temperature.

If the outer atmosphere is dry, the pressure due to the vapour of the liquid, actually present in the air will be low (b^1) and hence greater the evaporation. If the vapour of the liquid is removed as soon as it formed (under reduced pressure of vacuum), the space above the liquid does not become saturated with the vapour and evaporation proceeds faster.

Surface Area

From the above equation it is clear that the greater the surface area of the liquid, the greater will be the evaporation. Therefore, evaporators with larger heating surface area are preferred.

Moisture Content of the Feed

Many drugs undergoes hydrolysis readily in presence of moisture at high temperature. The decomposition is prevented by exposing the material to lower temperature and then exposed to higher temperature for final concentration. This method is used for preparation of dry extract of belladonna.

Type of Product Required

For evaporation, apparatus is selected based on type of product required. Open pan yields liquid or dry concentrate. Film evaporator produces liquid concentrate. Spray dryer produces products with good solubility. Vacuum evaporator gives porous product which are suitable for conversion to granules.

Time of Evaporation

If the constituents are thermostable, longer the time of exposure, greater will be the evaporation. It is well known that exposure of a drug to a relatively high temperature for a short period of time may cause less damage to active principles than a lower temperature with long exposure period. For this reason film evaporation are used.

Film and Deposits

When steam pan is used for concentration of vegetable extracts, a film may be formed on the surface of pan and precipitated matter may deposit on the heating surface. This film reduces the evaporating surface and transfer of heat diminished due to presence of precipitated matter. To avoid these problems efficient stirring is necessary.

Economic Factors

Economics of labour, fuel, floor space and materials are of important considerations. Considerable cost reduction takes place by the recovery of solvents and the utilization of *waste heat.*

For evaporation, heat is required to provide the latent heat of vaporization. Hence, rate of evaporation is controlled by rate of heat transfer. Therefore, evaporator is designed to give maximum heat transfer to the liquid.

EQUIPMENT

Steam Jacketed Kettle or Evaporating Pan

Principle: The aqueous extract is placed in a steam jacketed kettle (evaporating pan). The kettle is heated by the steam. The aqueous extract is heated by conduction and convection. The temperature increases and more solvent molecules escapes into vapour.

Construction: The construction of a steam jacketed kettle is shown in Fig. 5.1. It is hemispherical structure which consists of an inner pan called *kettle which* is enveloped with an outer pan called *jacket.* The two pans are joined to enclose a space through which steam is passed.

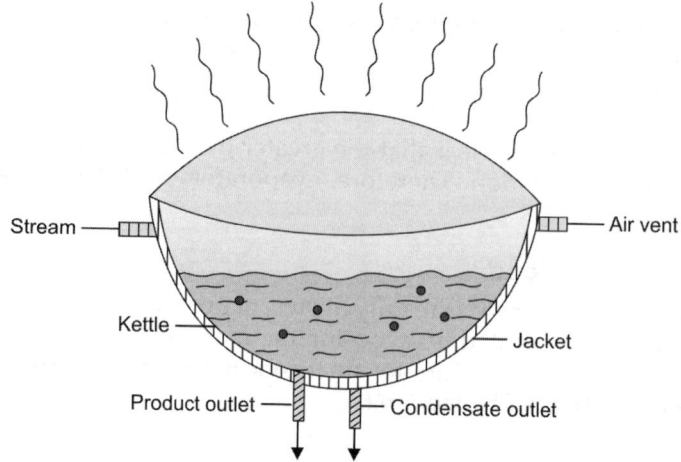

Fig. 5.1: Steam jacketed evaporator pan

For smaller quantities, kettle is made up of a single sheet of metal. For larger capacities, several sheets are welded. Kettle may be composed of copper is it is a suitable metal with good conductivity, though tinned copper is preferred as some amount of copper might dissolve if acidic materials are dissolved. An outlet for non condensed gases and an inlet for the steam is afforded near the top of the jacket. The outlet at the bottom vents the condensate whereas the product is discharged from the outlet at the bottom.

Working: Aqueous extract to be evaporated is placed in the kettle. Steam is supplied though the inlet. Contents are heated by the steam and the condensate leaves though the outlet. The contents are stirred manually for smaller volumes and mechanically for larger volumes. The rate of evaporation is fast in the initial stages and decreases gradually as the liquid gets concentrated.

Fans fitted over the pan not only remove the vapour and prevent condensation in the room, but also accelerate the rate of evaporation by removing saturated air from the surface of the liquid.

Uses: Evaporating pan is suitable for concentrating aqueous and thermostable liquids.

Advantages
- Evaporating pan is constructed both for small scale and large scale operations
- The equipment is simple in construction and easy to operate, clean and maintain
- The cost of installation and maintenance is low
- It can be constructed with copper, stainless steel and aluminum
- Removal of the product is easy.

Disadvantages
- Cost of production is more due to less heat economy
- Due to long-time of exposure, the equipment is not suitable for heat sensitive materials. As the product gets more concentrated, the heating area decreases
- It is open type of evaporator, presence of vapours into the atmosphere leads to saturation of the atmosphere which slows down the evaporation and also causes discomfort to operators
- Boiling point of water cannot be reduced, since reduced pressure cannot be created in open type evaporator.

Horizontal Tube Evaporator

Principle: In horizontal tube evaporator, steam is passed through the horizontal tubes, which are immersed in pool of liquid to be evaporated. Heat transfer takes place through the tubes heating the liquid outside the tubes. The solvent evaporates and escapes from the top of the evaporator. The concentrated liquid is collected from the bottom.

Construction: The construction of a horizontal tube evaporator is shown in Fig. 5.2. It consists of a large cylindrical body made up of cast iron or plate steel. An average size of the body ranges from 1.8 to 2.4 meters diameter and from 2.4 to 3.6 meter height.

The horizontal tube evaporator has a steam compartment with an inlet at one end for the steam in the lower part of the body. A vent is provided for the steam at the other end. At the bottom of the steam compartment, an outlet is provided for the condensate. About 6–8 horizontal stainless steel tubes are inserted in the steam compartment. The steam compartment width is about half the diameter of the body. There is provision for inlet for feed and outlet for vapour at the top of the dome. At the center of the conical bottom of the body, an other outlet for thick liquid is provided (Fig. 5.2). The feed is ushered into the evaporator to such a level that steam tubers are immersed in it. Steam is pushed into the steam compartment up to the horizontal tubes which conduct the steam to the liquid due to difference in temperature. The condensed steam passes through the outlet. The solvent is evaporated as the feed absorbs the heat. The vapours pass out through the outlet at the top. This process carried out until a thick liquid is formed. Up to the formation of thick liquid which can be collected from the bottom outlet.

Uses: Horizontal tube evaporator is used for non-viscous solution which does not deposit scales or crystals on evaporation.

Advantage: The cost per square meter of heating surface is usually less in horizontal tube evaporator.

Disadvantages

- It may be only used when rigorous boiling is obtained with natural circulation
- It cannot be used for viscous liquids
- It is difficult to clean.

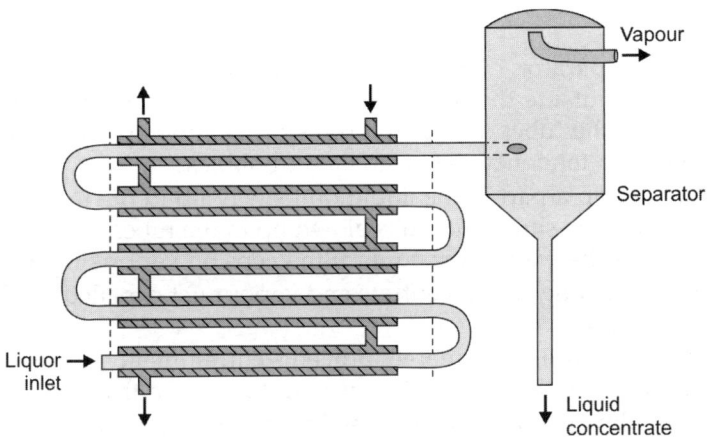

Fig. 5.2: Horizontal evaporator

CLIMBING FILM EVAPORATOR (RISING FILM EVAPORATOR)

Principle: In this type of evaporator tubes are heated externally by steam. The preheated feed enters from the bottom. The preheated feed entering from the bottom flows up via the heated tubes. The spiked overall coefficient of the preheated feed heats up the liquid quickly. The liquid near the wall converts into vapour and forms small bubbles which end up into large bubbles which progress further in the tubes along with entrapped slug. The liquid films from the top strike the deflector (entrainment separator) placed above which directs the liquid concentrate down to the lower part from where it is removed.

Construction: The construction of a climbing film evaporator is shown in Fig. 5.3. In this evaporator, the heating unit consists of steam jacketed tubes. The feed inlet is at the bottom of the steam compartment.

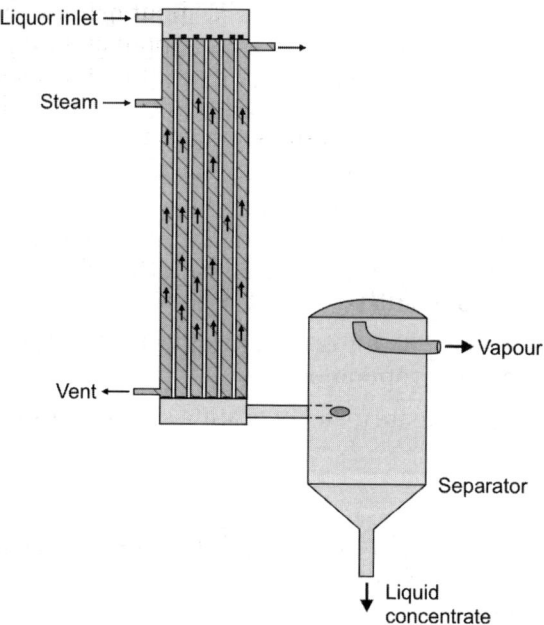

Fig. 5.3: Climbing film evaporator

An entrainment separator 1.2 meters above the tube at the bottom. Steam makes way into the spaces outside the tubes via the inlet. Heat is transferred to the liquid through the walls of the tubes. The liquid transforms into vapour and forms smaller bubbles, which have a tendency to fuse to larger bubbles.

These bubbles entrap a part of the liquid on its way up in the tubes. As additional vapours are formed, the slug of liquid is blown up in the tubes which help the liquid spread as a film over the walls. This liquid film keeps on vaporizing quickly.

Lastly, the mixture of liquid concentrate and vapour get expelled at a high velocity from the top of the tubes.

The entrainment separator not merely prevents entrainment, but also breaks foam. The vapour escapes from the top, while concentrate is taken from the bottom.

Uses: Climbing film evaporator can be used to concentrate thermolabile substances, such as insulin, liver extracts and vitamins.

Advantages

- Large area for heat transfer is provided by employing long and narrow tubes
- The heat transfer is enhanced as the resistance for heat transfer at the boundary layers is reduced due to flow of liquid at high velocity
- The time of contact between the liquor and the heating surface is very short. The liquid is in the heater for one second, while its residence time is 20 seconds in the evaporator. Hence, it is suitable for heat sensitive materials
- There is no elevation of boiling point due to hydrostatic head as the tubes are not submerged
- Presences of entrainment separator make it suitable for foam-forming liquids, because foam can be broken by an entrainment separator
- It requires small floor space.

Disadvantages

- Equipment is expensive, construction is quite complicated
- It is difficult to clean and maintain
- Large head space is required
- It is not advisable for very viscous liquids, salting liquids and scaling liquids
- If feed rate is high, the liquor may be concentrated insufficient. If feed rate is low, film cannot be maintained.

FORCED CIRCULATION EVAPORATOR

Principle: Forced circulation evaporators are similar to natural circular evaporators in principle, with the inclusion of mechanical agitators. In forced circulation evaporator, pump is used to circulate liquid through the tubes at high pressures. Forced circulation of the liquid also creates some form of agitation. There is a sudden drop in pressure when the liquid leaves the tubes and enters the vapour head which leads to the flashing of superheated liquor.

Construction: The construction of a forced circulation evaporator is shown in Fig. 5.4. The steam jacketed tubes are held between two tube sheets. The tube measures

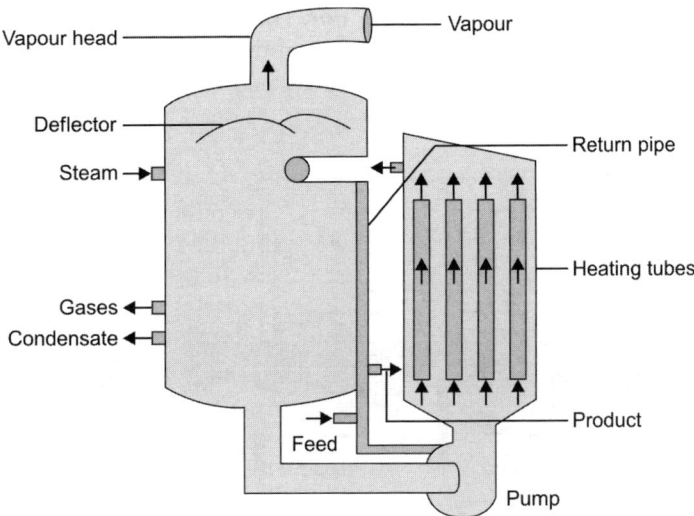

Fig. 5.4: Forced circulation evaporator

0.1 meter inside diameter and 2.5 meter long. The part of the tubes which projects into the vapour head (flash chamber) consists of a deflector. The vapour head is connected to a return pipe that runs downwards and enters into the inlet of a pump.

Working: In the forced circulation evaporator, liquid is pumped through the inside of a tubular heater at reasonably high velocities. Considerable coalescence of droplets occurs when liquid-vapour mixture is ejected from the tubes against a deflector. The shape of the deflector controls the entrainment from the evaporator. The liquid which is unevaporated is allowed to recirculate through an external piping arrangement to the pump which forces the liquid through the heating element. The external heating unit has considerable advantage in allowing greater ease of cleaning or replacement of tubes, improved average coefficient of heat transfer since, it is possible to install the heating element far below the liquid level in the vapour head to avoid boiling on the heating surface, greatly decreasing the rate of deposition of solids.

Uses: Forced circulation evaporator is suitable for thermolabile substances and is used for the concentration of insulin and liver extracts. The equipment is also suitable for crystallizing operations where crystals are to be suspended at all time.

Advantages

- Due to rapid liquid movement, the heat transfer coefficient is high
- Salting and scaling are not there because of rapid evaporation
- As pumping mechanism is used in this evaporator, making it suitable for high viscous preparations.

Disadvantage: In forced circulation evaporator, the hold-up of liquid is high. The equipment is expensive, because power (pump) is required for circulating the liquid.

MULTIPLE EFFECT EVAPORATORS

Vertical tube evaporators are connected in several ways so as to achieve large scale evaporation as well as greater economy. The multiple effect evaporators are not used in the pharmaceutical industry. The principles of multiple effect evaporators are explained using an example of triple effect evaporator with parallel feed mechanism.

Construction: The construction of a multiple effect evaporator is shown in Fig. 5.5 using 3 evaporators, i.e. triple effect evaporator. The vapour from evaporator one serves as a heating medium for the evaporator two. Similarly, vapour from evaporator two

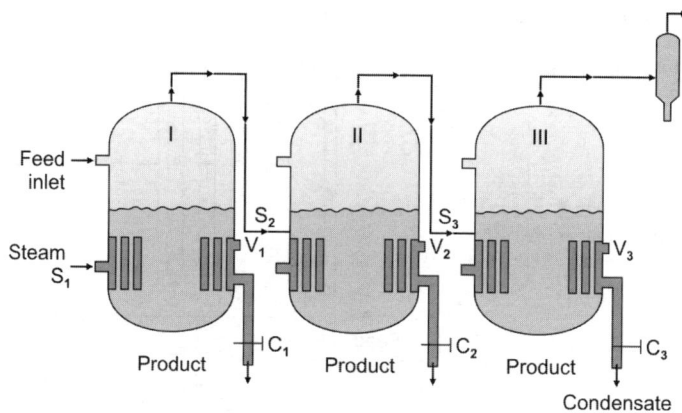

Fig. 5.5: Triple effect evaporator

serves as a heating medium for the evaporator three. Last evaporator is connected to a vacuum pump.

Working: Parallel feed arrangement is used in this example. A hot saturated solution of the feed is directly incorporated to each of the three effects (evaporation) simultaneously without transfering the material from one effect to the other. Salt solution is commonly concentrated by this method, in which the solute gets crystallized on concentration without increasing the viscosity.

Operations: At the start, the equipment is kept at room temperature and atmospheric pressure. The liquid feed is inserted to all the three evaporators up to the level of the upper tube sheets. The following operations are performed to achieve the effects as specified below.

- The vent valves V_1, V_2 and V_3 remain open while all other valves are closed
- Then a high vacuum is generated in the liquid chambers of evaporators
- The steam valves S_1 and condensate valve C_1 are opened. Then steam is fed. Steam initially replaces cold air from steam space of evaporator one. The valve, V_1 is stopped when all the cold air is purged
- Steam is constantly fed until the desired pressure P_0 is produced in the steam space of evaporator one. At this pressure, the temperature of the steam is t_0
- Steam transfers its heat to the liquid feed in the evaporator one and is condensed. Condensate is collected through the valve C_1
- The liquid temperature increases due to heat transfer and reaches the boiling point and vapour will be generated from the liquid feed
- These vapour displaces air in the upper part of evaporator one. The vapour also displaces the air in the steam space of the evaporator two
- The valve V_2 is closed after complete displacement of air by vapour in the steam compartment of evaporator two
- The vapour of evaporator one transfers its heat to the liquid of evaporator two and gets condensed. Condensate is removed through the valve C_2. These steps are repeated in the evaporator three.

As the liquid in the evaporator one gains heat, it reduces the difference in temperatures between the liquid and steam with a reduction in the rate of condensation. The temperature of the liquid in evaporator 1 is increased to its boiling point t_1 which gradually increases the pressure in the vapour space of evaporator one to P_1 and the temperature difference $(t_0 - t_1)$ is decreased.

Same changes occur in the evaporator 2 as the liquid reaches the boiling point. Likewise, the process is repeated in evaporator 3. Ultimately, three evaporators come to a stable state as the liquid boils in all the three effects one reduces. To maintain the liquid level constant, feed is introduced through the feed valve. Similarly evaporation of liquid takes place in evaporators two and three. Feed valves F_2 and F_3 are used for evaporators two and three respectively to maintain liquid levels constant. This process is continued until the liquid in all the evaporators attained the desired viscosity.

Then a thick liquid is collected by opening the product valves. Therefore, in this evaporator, there is a continuous supply of feed, steam and continuous withdrawal of liquid from all the three evaporators. Evaporator operates continuously with all the temperatures and pressures in balance.

The method of introduction of feed varies in this evaporators, it can be by forward feed method, backward feed method and mixed feed method. In the forward feed method, the mother liquor is introduced into evaporator one, then transferred to evaporator two and then to evaporator three. In the backward feed method, the mother liquor is first introduced into the evaporator three, then transferred to evaporator two and then transferred to evaporator one. In mixed feed method, the mother liquor is introduced into evaporator two then transferred to evaporator three and then transferred to evaporator one.

Uses

- It is used for product concentration
- It helps in solvent recovery
- It is used in various industries, such as sugar juice concentration, water recycling from distillery effluent, process evaporators, pharma, dye stuff, polymers, paint and other process industries.

Advantages

- It is suitable for large scale and for continuous operation
- It is highly economical compared to single effect
- About 5 evaporators can be attached.

Disadvantages

- The product can be backing up in the evaporator due to choking
- The evaporator body is heavily scaled
- The feed rate is excessive
- Large space required.

ECONOMY OF MULTIPLE EFFECT EVAPORATORS

The economy of an evaporator is the quantity of vapour produced per unit steam admitted. It is calculated by considering the following assumptions:

Feed is introduced at its boiling point. Hence, any more heat is not required to raise its temperature. The supplied steam gets condensed to give heat of condensation. This heat will then be transferred completely to the liquid and it then serves as latent heat of vaporization, i.e. liquid undergoes vaporization by receiving heat. Heat loss nevertheless is negligible.

The economy of an evaporator is expressed as:

Economy of an evaporator = Total mass of vapour produced = Total mass of steam supplied.

In single effect evaporator, steam generates vapour only once. Hence economy of a single effect evaporator = N units of vapour produced = 1 N units of steam.

In multiple effect evaporator, one unit of steam generates vapour many times, depending on the number of evaporators linked. Hence,

Economy of a multiple effect evaporator = N units of vapour produced = N 1 units of steam.

Therefore, economy of multiple effect evaporator is N times the economy of the single effect evaporator.

However, such a great economy is approximately true as it depends on many factors, such as temperature of the feed, temperature range in the evaporator, ratio of weight offered to the product and pressure difference.

VERY SHORT QUESTIONS

1. Define the term evaporation and state its applications.
2. Explain evaporation in terms of capacity and economy as applied to evaporation practice.
3. Describe the construction of calandria. Give its uses.
4. How many effects generally go into a multiple effect evaporator?
5. Explain advantages and uses of evaporating pan.

SHORT QUESTIONS

1. Elaborate the concept of multiple effect evaporation. What specific advantage does it offer?
2. Describe the construction, working, merits and demerits of climbing film evaporator.
3. Explain the construction and working of a forced circulation evaporator.
4. What do you understand by economy of multiple effect evaporator?
5. Give detail account on horizontal tube evaporator.

LONG QUESTIONS

1. How do film evaporator function? Elaborate the answer with a neat sketch of one such evaporator. List the merits and demerits of film evaporator system.
2. Classify evaporators. Describe construction and working of a steam jacketed kettle.
3. Explain the terms 'multiple effect evaporator' and 'evaporator capacity'.
4. Describe one such evaporator. How do you feed such evaporator?
5. Explain factors affecting evaporation and elaborate its objectives.

MULTIPLE CHOICE QUESTIONS

1. Evaporation takes place at:
   a. Freezing point
   b. Boiling point
   c. In-between freezing point and boiling point
   d. At all temperatures

2. .... is not an assumption in the evaporator model?
   a. The feed has only one volatile components
   b. Only the latent heat of vaporization is available for heating the solution
   c. Boiling action in heat exchanger ensures perfect mixing
   d. Overall temperature driving force is the temperature of saturated steam

3. **Larger the surface area of liquid then evaporation will be:**
   a. Small   b. Large
   c. Moderate   d. None of above

4. **Change of liquid into vapours from surface of liquid without heating is known as:**
   a. Expansion   b. Contraction
   c. Evaporation   d. Fusion

5. **Evaporation from surface of any liquid depends on:**
   a. Temperature   b. Wind
   c. Nature of liquid   d. All of above

6. **Evaporation causes:**
   a. Cooling   b. Heating effect
   c. Increase in weight   d. Increase in density

7. **Among the following is a characteristic of a horizontal tube evaporator?**
   a. Agitation is provided only by bubbles leaving the evaporator as vapour
   b. The tube bundle is arranged vertically, with the solution inside the tubes condensing outside
   c. To handle viscous solution a pump is used to force liquid upwards
   d. Also called short vertical tube evaporator

8. **.................. process used to obtain the solute from the solution is called:**
   a. Evaporation   b. Distillation
   c. Condensation   d. None of above

9. **Answer which statement is true or false:**
   1. Evaporation is considered a mass and heat transfer operation.
   2. After evaporation, solids are left behind.
   a. True, False   b. True, True
   c. False, False   d. False, True

10. **In evaporation of edible solutions, the BPR-boiling point rise should be .... and the foaming and scale formation should be ....**
    a. Low, minimum
    b. High, maximum
    c. Low, maximum
    d. High, minimum

11. **Which of the following is true while concentrating jams?**
    a. They are sensitive to heat
    b. Evaporation process for jams is carried out under vacuum
    c. At vacuum, the boiling point decreases
    d. All of the mentioned

12. **Which statement is true or false?**
    1. Boiling point rise is due to the colligative properties due to the presence of solid particles in the solvent.

2. Boiling point rise is due to the increase in pressure at the bottom of the solvent due to hydrostatic head of the column.

a. True, False
b. True, True
c. False, False
d. False, True

13. **Pick the correct statement:**

a. Duhring's rule states that the ratio of temperatures at which two solutions have the same vapour pressure is a constant

b. Duhring's rule states that the boiling point of a solution is a linear function of the boiling point of pure water at the same pressure

c. Both a and b

d. None of above

14. **What is the total mass of water vaporized per unit mass of steam input to the evaporator.**

a. Efficiency of evaporator
b. Economy of evaporator
c. Rate of evaporator
d. Capacity of evaporator

15. **State true or false. Single effect evaporation is simple and steam effective.**

a. True

b. False

16. .... **is often used to compare a pure liquid and a solution at a given concentration.**

a. Duhring's rule
b. Plank rule
c. Friction rule
d. Doppler rule

17. **Evaporator that is used to natural circulation is:**

a. Horizontal tube evaporator

b. Vertical tube evaporator

c. Vacuum pan evaporator

d. Forced circulation evaporator

18. **Name the evaporators in which pumps are used to force the evaporating liquid through the tubes are:**

a. Horizontal tube evaporator

b. Vertical tube evaporator

c. Vacuum pan evaporator

d. Forced circulation evaporator

19. .... **consists of one pass vertical shell and tube heat exchanger discharging the product to be evaporated into a relatively small vapor head?**

a. Horizontal tube evaporator

b. Long tube vertical evaporator

c. Vacuum pan evaporator

d. Forced circulation evaporator

Distillation

Jayamanti Pandit and Yasmin Sultana

Distillation is a process defined as the separation of the constituents of a mixture by boiling the liquid mixture and collecting the vapour as condensate. Such separation may include:

- Separation of liquid from non-volatile impurities
- Separation of one liquid from one or more other liquids with which it may be miscible, partially miscible or immiscible.

The process is based on the principle of relative volatility or boiling points.

Volatility is a measure of the tendency of substance to vaporize. Relative volatility is a measure of vapour pressures of the components in a liquid mixture. It is easy to separate if the liquid have widely different volatility.

When heat is applied, temperature of the liquid increases up to certain temperature which is called the boiling point beyond this temperature if additional heat is applied causes the vaporization of that liquid. The boiling point is physical and characteristic property for identification of the substance.

Hence, the process of distillation is heating a substance until it vaporizes, cooling the vapours, and collecting the condensed liquid.

THEORY APPLIED TO BINARY MIXTURES

Binary mixtures are those in which two liquids may be miscible with each other in all proportion, e.g. ethanol—water, acetone—water, benzene—carbon tetrachloride. On the basis of degree of miscibility of two liquids, these systems are classified as follows:

1. Completely miscible liquids
2. Partially miscible liquids
3. Immiscible liquids

Completely Miscible Liquids

Ideal solutions: An ideal solution obeys **Raoult's law**. It states that the partial pressure exerted by each component is proportional to its molar concentration in the solution. The law may be expressed by equation

$$P = p_A + p_B = p_A^0 X_A + p_B^0 X_B$$

where p is the total vapour pressure above a liquid mixture containing X_A and X_B mole fractions of component A and B, respectively, p_A^0 and p_B^0 are the vapour pressure exerted by the pure components, and p_A and p_B are the partial vapour pressure exerted by the components in the liquid mixture. The components of ideal solutions have a similar chemical structure, e.g. benzene and toluene, n-hexane and n-heptane, ethyl bromide and ethyl iodide.

The partial pressure of each component in an ideal solution p_A and p_B and composition of solution at constant temperature are plotted graphically (Fig. 6.1), where $O_A p_A^0$ and $O_B p_B^0$ indicate the variations in partial pressures exerted by component A and B. It can be shown that the line $p_A^0 p_B^0$ will indicate the variation in total vapour pressure with composition.

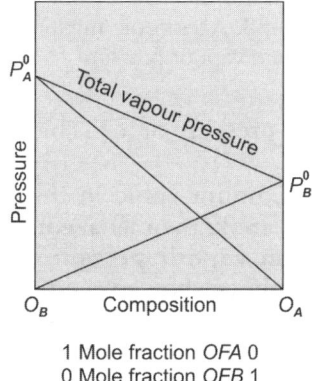

Fig. 6.1: Vapour-composition diagram for an ideal solution

1 Mole fraction OFA 0
0 Mole fraction OFB 1

Real solutions: Depending on the nature of liquids and temperature, liquid-liquid systems showed deviation from Raoult's law.

Negative deviation from Raoult's law: When interactions, such as hydration, hydrogen bonding, or salt formation occurs between the components of a solution, then the vapour pressure of each component is lowered with respect to an ideal solution and the system is said to exhibits a negative deviation from Raoult's law, e.g. chloroform and acetone, pyridine and acetic acid, water and nitric acid.

Posititve deviation from Raoult's law: Vapour pressures of most of the systems are greater than those of an ideal solution and such system exhibits a positive deviation from Raoult's law. It occurs when the components shows differences in their polarity, degree of association and length of hydrocarbon chain, e.g. carbon tetrachloride and cyclohexane, benzene and ethanol, water and ethanol. In this the degree of deviation from Raoult's law decreases as the temperature increases.

The solutions of liquids in liquids are classified into three types based on their deviation from ideal behaviour:

1. Systems in which the total vapour pressure is always intermediate between those of the pure components. It means that there is neither a minimum nor a maximum in the vapour pressure-composition diagram (Fig. 6.2A). These type of systems are known as **zeotropic mixture**, e.g. water-methanol, carbon tetrachloride-cyclohexane.

2. Systems that exhibit a minimum value in the vapour pressure composition diagram (Fig. 6.2B). These are called **azeotropic mixtures with a maximum boiling**

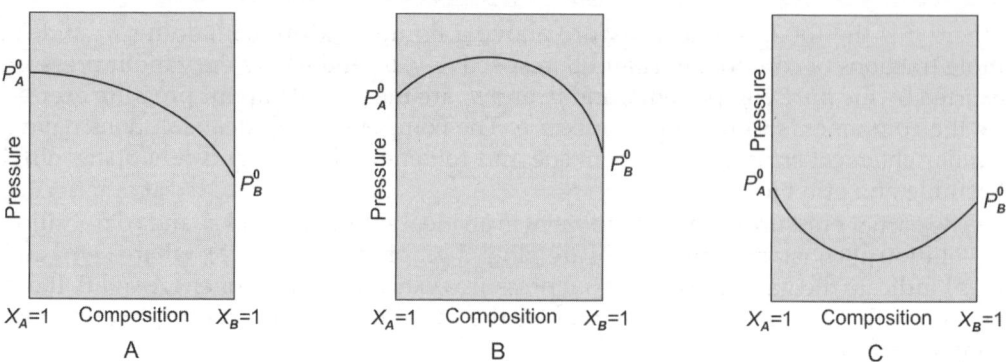

Figs 6.2A to C: Effect of deviation from ideal behaviour on total vapour pressure of various liquid mixtures: A. Zeotropic mixture; B. Azeotropic mixture with a maximum vapour pressure; C. Azeotropic mixture with a minimum vapour pressure.

point or minimum vapour pressure or, e.g. chloroform-acetone, pyridine-acetic acid, water-nitric acid.

3. Systems that exhibit a maximum value in the vapour pressure-composition diagram (Fig. 6.3A). These are known as **azeotropic mixture with a** minimum boiling point or **maximum vapour pressure**, e.g. benzene-ethanol, water-ethanol. Figures 6.3A to C above showed the relation between vapour pressure and composition of the liquid phase. If these diagrams are drawn to show the variation in vapour pressure with both vapour and liquid compositions, Figs 6.3A to C.

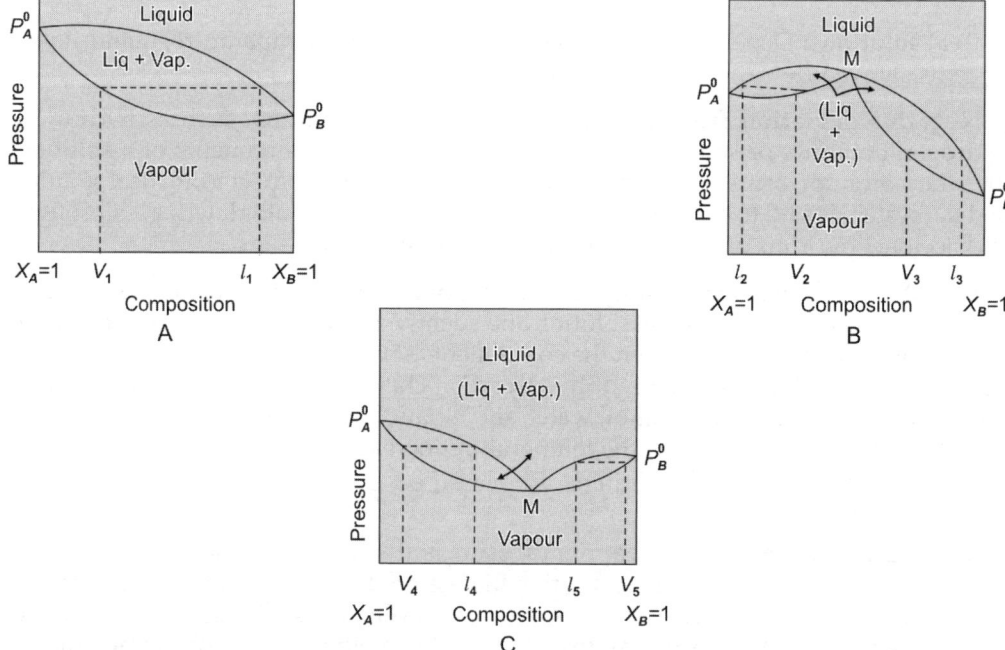

Figs 6.3A to C: Vapour pressure diagrams showing liquid and vapour composition curves for various liquids mixtures: A. Zeotropic mixture; B. Azeotropic mixture with a maximum vapour pressure; C. Azeotropic mixture with a minimum vapour pressure

In Figs 6.3A to C, the upper curves represent the variation in total vapour pressure with composition of the liquid phase and lower curve represent the variation in total vapour pressure with composition of the vapour phase. The vapour phase in equilibrium with a particular liquid composition is richer in more volatile component A; i.e. the component with the higher vapour pressure (Fig. 6.3A). This is known as **Konowaloff's Rule**. The point M corresponds to the formation of an azeotrope, which is a mixture with a lower or higher vapour pressure than is exerted by any other composition in the system (Figs 6.3B and C). This is the point where the compositions of vapour and liquid are identical.

Partially Miscible Liquids

a. *Systems showing an increase in miscibility with rise in temperature*

Due to difference in the cohesive forces between the molecules of each component in a liquid mixture, a positive deviation from Raoult's law arises. As the temperature decreases this difference becomes more marked and the positive deviation results in decrease in miscibility which is sufficient to cause the separation of the mixture into two phases. A saturated solution of one more phenol is added, and then a second layer separates. This is a saturated solution of water in liquid phenol. The line DC in the curve represents the effect of temperature on the solubility of water in phenol. On further addition of phenol, an unsaturated solution of water in phenol is produced. It can be seen from the curve that BC and DC meets at C; above C only one liquid phase can exist. The two components are miscible in all proportions above C, which is known as the upper critical temperature (upper CST).

b. *Systems showing a decrease in miscibility with rise in temperature.*

A few mixtures show a lower critical solution temperature (lower CST), e.g. triethylamine plus water, paraldehyde plus water. These mixture involves the formation of a compound that causes a negative deviation from Raoult's law. As the temperature decreases, miscibility increases.

c. *Systems showing upper and lower CST*

The decrease in miscibility with increase in temperature in systems having a lower CST is not indefinite. Above certain temperature, positive deviation from Raoult's law become important and with rise in temperature, miscibility increase again.

Effect of Added Substances on CST

CST is very sensitive to added substances or impurities. Blending is the term used for the addition of a third substance to increase the miscibility of two liquids. This is applied in the preparation of cresol with soap solution. Cresol is partially miscible with water; addition of soap decreases the upper CST and produces complete miscibility at ordinary temperatures.

Immiscible Liquids

In a mixture containing two immiscible liquids each liquid exerts its own vapour pressure independently of another. The total vapour pressure (p), is the sum of the all vapour pressures separately, of the pure compounds, i.e.

$$p = p^0A + p^0B$$

The liquid mixture will boil when its total vapour pressure is comes out to be equal to the atmospheric pressure. It shows that the boiling point of the mixture is lower than that of either of the pure component.

If ideal behaviour occurs, the constant boiling mixture will produce a vapour in which the number of molecules of each component is proportional to its vapour pressure.

$$\frac{nA}{nB} = \frac{p^0 A}{p^0 B}$$

But, $n_A = m_A/M_A$ and $n_B = m_B/M_B$

where, m_A and m_B are the masses of each component in the vapour and M_A and M_B are their molecular weights

From the above equations, $m_A/M_A \times M_B/m_B = p_A^0/p_B^0$

$$m_A/m_B = p_A^0 \, M_A/p_B^0 \, M_B$$

This equation indicates that the ratio of A to B by weight in the distillate is proportional to the ratios of their partial pressures and their molecular weights. Thus if an immiscible mixture of an organic compound and water is distilled, a high proportion of the distillate will be comprised of the organic compound, since water has a low molecular weight. This process is known as **steam distillation**. Steam distillation is used as a means to purify organic compounds which do not react and are immiscible with water.

Steam distillation is used for extracting most of the volatile oils, such as clove, anise and eucalyptus. It is used for purification of high boiling point fixed oil, e.g. essential oil of almond. This method is used for separation of two immiscible liquids, preparation of aromatic waters and distillation of camphor.

Phase Equilibria

Phase equilibria is the equilibrium between the phases solid, liquid and gas.

The phase rule: It is an expression of the conditions relating to physical equilibria between various states of matter. A phase is defined as any homogenous and physically distinct part of a system that is separated from other parts of the system by definite boundaries. For example, a mixture of gases always constitute one phase because the mixture is homogenous and there are no bounding surfaces between the gases. But, ice, water and water vapour are three separated phases; they are distinct phases and there are definite boundaries between them.

The number of components of a system is the smallest number of independent chemical constituents necessary to express the concentration of all phases present in the system, e.g. in the three phase system of ice, water and water vapour, the number of component is one, since each phase can be expressed in terms of H_2O.

The number of degrees of freedom is the number of variable conditions, such as temperature, pressure, and concentration that is necessary to state in order that it is necessary to state in order that the conditions of the system at equilibrium may be completely defined.

The relationship between the number of phases, P, components, C, and degrees of freedom, F, for equilibria that are influenced only by temperature, pressure and concentration is given by the following equation, which is the quantitative expression of the phase rule.

$$F = C - P + 2$$

Phase diagrams: The effects of temperature, pressure and composition on the phase equilibria will be indicated by graphs called **phase diagrams**, which shows a variation of a transition temperature such as a boiling point or a melting point with pressure or composition.

Volatility and relative volatility: The **volatility** in a liquid solution of any substance is defined as the equilibrium partial pressure of the substance in vapour phase divided by the mole fraction of the substance in a liquid solution.

Volatility of component a in a liquid solution $= V_a = P_a/X_a$

where, P_a and X_a are the partial pressure and mole fraction of a component respectively.

The volatility of a material in its pure state is equal to the vapour pressure exerted by the material itself in the pure state while the volatility of a component in a liquid mixture which follows Raoult's law must be equal to the vapour pressure of that component in the pure state.

Relative volatility is a measure of the difference in volatility between two components, and hence their boiling points. It indicates the easy of separation of a component from the mixture. The relative volatility (α), which may be defined as ratio of the volatility of the components in the liquid mixture. Usually relative volatilities are expressed in the numerator with the higher of the two volatilities.

$$\alpha_{ab} = V_a/V_b = P_a X_b/P_b X_a$$

If the relative volatility between two components is very close to one, it indicates that they have similar vapour pressure characteristics and boiling points and thus it will be very difficult to separate the two components via distillation.

If the components follow Raoult's law,

$$P_a = P_a^0 X_a$$
$$P_b = P_b^0 X_b$$

P_b^0 is the vapour pressure. Combine Raoult's law with the relative volatility to get:

$$\alpha_{ab} = P_a^0/P_b^0$$

This means the relative volatility is the ratio of vapour pressures. Relative volatility is useful for designing all type of distillation processes and separations that involves the contacting of vapour and liquid phases in a series of equilibrium stages.

An increase in pressure and temperature has a significant effect on the relative volatility of the components in a liquid mixture. Since both affect each other.

Boiling point diagrams: The boiling point diagram gives the equilibrium compositions of the components in a liquid mixture at various temperatures with a fixed pressure. Consider an example of binary mixture containing two components A and B. The boiling point of A is that at which the mole fraction of A is 1 and more volatile (lower boiling point than B) component. The boiling point of B is that at which the mole fraction of A is 0.

The upper curve in the diagram is called the dew-point curve while the lower one is called the bubble-point curve. The dew-point is defined as the temperature at which when the saturated vapour starts to condense while bubble-point is that temperature at which the liquid starts to boil. The region below the bubble-point curve shows the equilibrium composition of the sub-cooled liquid whereas the region above the dew-point in a curve shows the equilibrium composition of the superheated vapour.

This difference between liquid and vapour compositions is the basis for distillation operations. The boiling point diagrams for various liquid mixtures are discussed below.

Zeotropic Mixtures

A boiling point diagram for a zeotropic mixture (which shows the variation in boiling point with composition of the liquid and vapour phases at constant pressure) is used to explain the effects of distillation on this liquid system. In Fig. 6.4, upper and lower curves represent the vapour composition and the liquid composition respectively and the areas corresponding to liquid and vapour phases are transposed when compared with the vapour pressure diagram (Fig. 6.3A). On applying Konowaloff's rule to boiling point diagram, it is seen that a liquid with a composition corresponding to l_1 will boil at temperature T_1 and is in equilibrium with vapours of composition l_2. This vapour is richer in component A, which has a lower boiling point (T_A) and is the more volatile component of the liquid mixture. If the vapour of composition l_2 is removed and condensed, liquid of composition l_2 is obtained. On heating this liquid at temperature T_2, a vapour of composition l_3 is obtained which is richer in component A, i.e. the composition of the distillate will approach closer to pure A as more stages of heating and condensation are involved. As the component A is distilled over, the component B gradually increases in the flask. Thus fractional distillation can be employed to completely separate the components of a zeotropic mixture by a series of vaporization and condensation cycles in a distillation column.

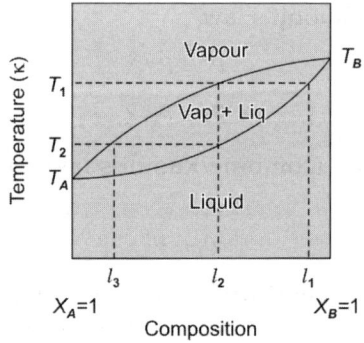

Fig. 6.4: Boiling point composition diagram for a zeotropic system

Azeotropic Mixture with a Maximum Boiling Point

The boiling point diagram for such type of system is represented by Fig. 6.5A. Irrespective of the initial composition of the liquid mixture, complete separation into pure A and pure B cannot be achieved. This is due to coincident liquid and vapour composition curves at point M. A liquid with a composition corresponding to this point boils at a maximum temperature for the system and produces a vapour with the same composition. These mixtures can be separated into pure A or pure B as distillate and a constant boiling mixture of composition M which remains in the distillation flask. The nature of the distillate (i.e. A or B) will depends on the composition of the initial mixture with respect to that of the constant boiling azeotrope.

Azeotropic Mixtures with a Minimum Boiling Point

The boiling point diagram for this type of system is shown in Fig. 6.5B. Fractional distillation of this type of mixtures will allow separation of the mixture into pure A or pure B only, and a constant boiling mixture with a composition corresponding to M. Pure A or B will remain in the distillation flask after the constant boiling mixture has been removed completely at a minimum boiling point. The nature of the pure liquid obtained in the flask (i.e. A or B) will depends on the composition of the initial mixture with respect to constant boiling azeotrope.

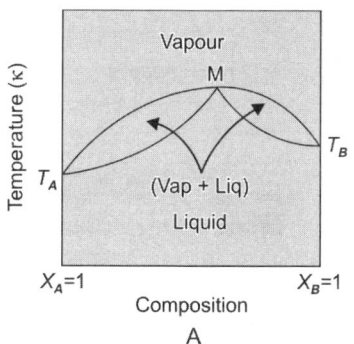 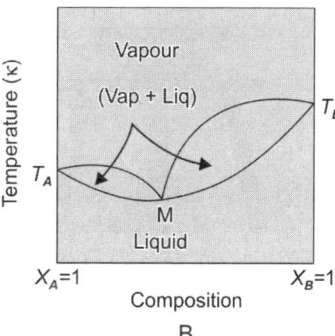

Figs 6.5A and B: Boiling point composition diagram for azeotropic mixtrues: A. Maximum boiling poing areotropes; B. Minimum boiling point azeotrope

TYPES OF DISTILLATION

Simple Distillation

It is a process of converting a single constituent liquid (or mixture) into its vapour and transfer the vapour to another place thus, recovering the liquid by condensing the vapour as it comes into contact with a cold surface. It can be conducted in two ways (1) Equilibrium vaporization or Flash distillation (2) Differential distillation.

Principle: Simple distillation is conducted at its boiling point. Liquid boils when its vapour pressure is equal to the atmospheric pressure. The higher the relative volatility of a liquid, the better is the separation by simple distillation. Heat is supplied to the liquid so that it boils. The resulting vapour is transferred to a different place and condensed. Simple distillation is a useful method of purification and separation if the liquid is volatile and remaining components are non volatile.

Applications

- It is used in the preparation of distilled water and water for injection
- This method is used for the purification of organic solvents and preparation of aromatic waters. Aromatic spirit of ammonia and spirit of nitrous ether are a few official compounds which are prepared by this method
- Non-volatile solids can be separated from volatile liquids.

Laboratory Scale Apparatus Based on Simple Distillation

Construction: The construction is shown in Fig. 6.6 consisting of distillation flask to carry the separating mixture. It has a side arm sloping downward and fitted to a condenser by means of a cork. The condenser is attached to a receiving flask by using an adapter. The apparatus is completely made of glass.

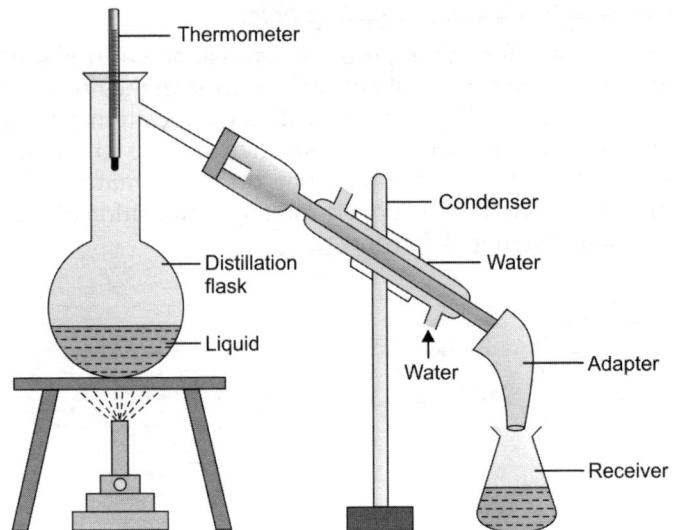

Fig. 6.6: Laboratory scale of simple distillation

Working: The liquid which is required to be distilled is filled and put into the flask to at least one-half to two-thirds of its volume. A small piece of porcelain or porous pot must be added in the distillation flask before distillation to avoid boiling bumping of the liquid. A thermometer is inserted to check the temperature inside the flask. The thermometer must be adjusted just below the side arm through a cork fitted to the flask. Cold water is circulated through the jacket of the condenser.

The content in the flask are heated and the vapours of the boiling liquid begin to rise up and enter into the condenser in the side arm. The vapours in the condenser get condensed and collected into the receiving flask. The flame must adjust so that one to two drops of condensed liquid is collected per seconds. The distillation must be continued till a small volume of liquid remains in the flask.

Steam Distillation

Steam distillation is used to separate two miscible liquids which are highly heat sensitive or decompose below their boiling point like essential oils. For example, the substances which are insoluble in water and decompose by heat can be separated by steam.

Principle

A mixture of liquids began to boil when the vapour pressure of the liquid is equal to the surrounding pressure. Boiling point is pressure dependent phenomena and it increases if the surrounding pressure increases and vice versa. For example, a liquid X decomposes at 50°C and it has normal boiling point of 70°C at atmospheric pressure. If we have to separate liquid X from water at 1 atm, in normal condition it is not possible because liquid X will decompose at 50°C before it reaches to 70°C, its boiling point to overcome such problem steam distillation is used and applicable to separate such mixture where the component is heat sensitive and decompose below boiling point.

Steam is used to boil the liquid mixture and this steam is able to provide gentle heating to vaporise the heat sensitive component without decomposition. It is not suitable for immiscible liquid which reacts with water.

Equipment

Construction: Simple laboratory steam distillation equipment assembly is shown in Fig. 6.7. It consists of metallic can fitted with a cork having entry for two tubes on hole. Larger tube is passed through the first hole as to reach the bottom of the steam. The tube is known as safety tube so that, if the pressure inside the steam generator is high the water will force steam out of it and pressure will be reduced. Through 2nd hole, a bend tube is passed in order to connect them with the flask containing non aqueous liquid through a rubber bung. This tube also reaches the bottom of the flask. Another delivery tube is inserted through the other hole of the rubber bung which connects the flask with the condenser. This condenser is further connected to a receiver using an adaptor.

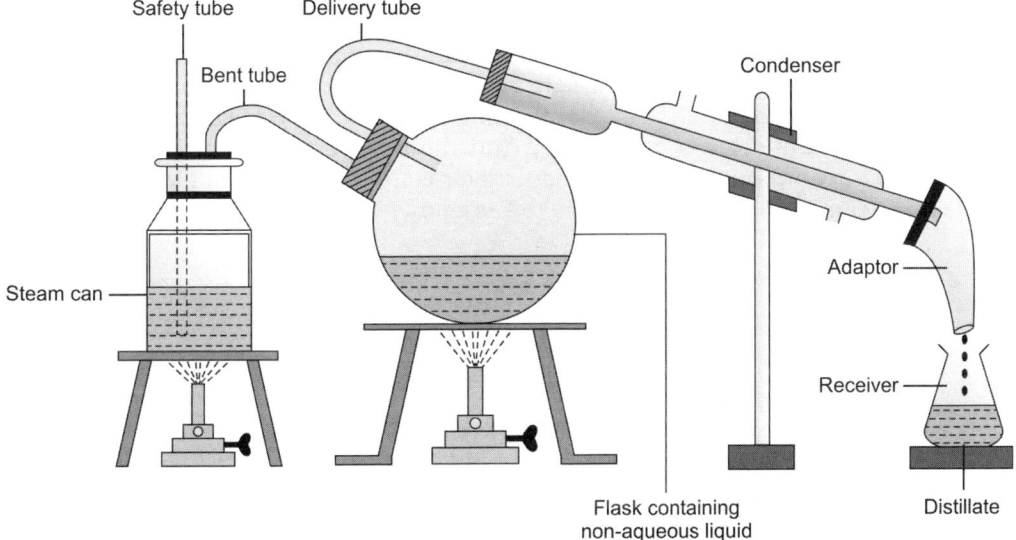

Fig. 6.7: Steam distillation

Working: The non-aqueous liquid placed in the flask is mixed with small quantity of water. Water is filled in the steam can and heated. When steam generated from steam flask is passed through the boiling mixture. The non-aqueous liquid mixture heat up and the steam carrying volatile fraction will pass into the condenser where it gets cooled and collected into the receiver. The receiver may contain water and organic liquid which can be separated by using a separating flask.

Applications

- It is employed for extraction and purification of essential oils
- Volatile oils from plants, such as clove, anise, eucalyptus, etc. are also manufactured by steam distillation
- It is useful for separating immiscible liquid at lower temperature than the boiling point
- Steam distillation is used in the preparation of aromatic water and perfumes.

Distillation Under Reduced Pressure

It is the distillation process in which the liquid is distilled by the application of vacuum at a temperature lower than its boiling point. It is a modification of simple distillation process, wherein vacuum pumps and suction pumps are used to reduce the pressure.

Boiling occurs when the vapour pressure is equal to atmospheric pressure and if the pressure is reduced by application of vacuum the liquid boils at a lower temperature and boiling point of the liquid gets lowered.

Vacuum distillation

It is a method of distillation where the pressure at which the liquid mixture to be distilled is reduced to less than its vapour pressure, i.e. usually less than the atmospheric pressure causing evaporation of most volatile liquids. It works on the principle that boiling of a liquid occurs when the vapour pressure exceeds the ambient pressure. It can be used with or without heating the mixture. It is also known as low temperature distillation.

Construction: The distillation unit consists of a claisen flask, i.e. a double neck distillation flask, a condenser, a receiver, vacuum pump and a thermometer which is fitted in one of the neck of claisen flask. In another neck of claisen flask, a fine capillary tube is inserted which would prevent bumping of liquid. This claisen flask through a condenser gets connected to a receiver. And the receiver is connected through an adapter to a vacuum pump. A small manometer is inserted between the receiver and the vacuum pump. Figure 6.8 illustrate the assembly of vacuum distillation.

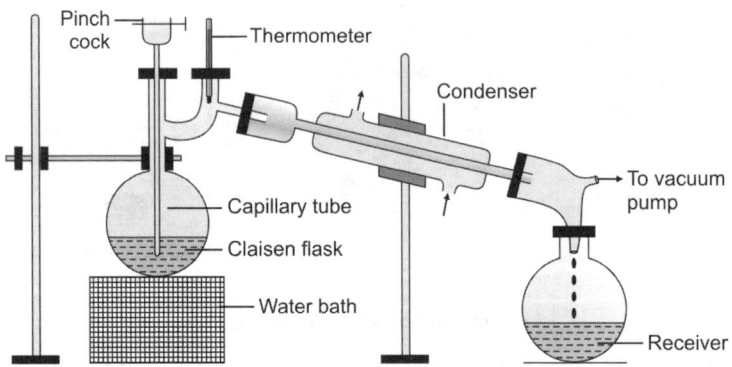

Fig. 6.8: Distillation under reduced pressure

Working: In operation, the flask is filled up with half to one-third of volume of liquid to be distilled. In the claisen flask the capillary tube and thermometer are placed. Under the application of vacuum the contents of flask are gradually heated. Due to vacuum the temperature rises and liquid gets rapidly vaporized. Through the condenser the vapour passes and the condensate is collected in a receiver.

Applications

- It is used for liquid having low boiling points or chemically unstable at their atmospheric boiling points
- Vacuum distillation is the method of choice to remove solvents from the temperature sensitive mixture without changing the product
- There is a lower level of residue build-up as compared to steam distillation. At industrial scale, a dry vacuum distillation column is used in oil refineries.

Advantages

- It increases the relative volatility of the key components making more effective separation of the two components

- It reduces the temperature requirement as the process is done under reduced pressure. This is useful for the products which degrade or polymerize at elevated temperature
- The separated products have high yield and purity.

Flash Distillation (or Equilibrium Vaporization)

It is a continuous process where the liquid mixture suddenly vaporizes while passing through a high pressure zone to a low pressure zone. It is also known as equilibrium distillation because the separation will take place only when the liquid has and vapour phase comes in equilibrium.

Principle: When a heated liquid mixture enters from a high pressure area to a low pressure zone the liquid mixture gets instantly vaporized.

This process of instant vaporization is called flash vaporization. The chamber gets cooled and the molecules of the vapour phase with high boiling fraction turns to condensed, while the low boiling fraction remains as vapour. The liquid and vapour are in intimate contact for sufficient length of time so that equilibrium is reached. The liquid and vapours are separated and vapour is allowed to condense.

Construction: It consists of a pump, which is connected to a feed reservoir. Pump helps in pumping the feed into the heating chamber which contains a suitable heating mechanism. The heating chamber is connected to the vapour liquid separator through a reducing valve. The vapour outlet is at the top of vapour separator while liquid outlet is provided at the bottom as shown in Fig. 6.9.

Working: The feed is pumped into the heating chamber at a certain pressure. The heated liquid gets enter through a pressure reducing valve into the vapour-liquid separator. The vaporization process is enhanced due to decrease in pressure. Cooling is produced due to sudden vaporization. The low boiling fractions remains as vapour while the vapour phase molecules of high boiling fraction get condensed. The vapour liquid mixture is kept in contact for a sufficient length of time so that equilibrium is achieved. The vapour is collected at top of the separator and liquid is separated from the bottom.

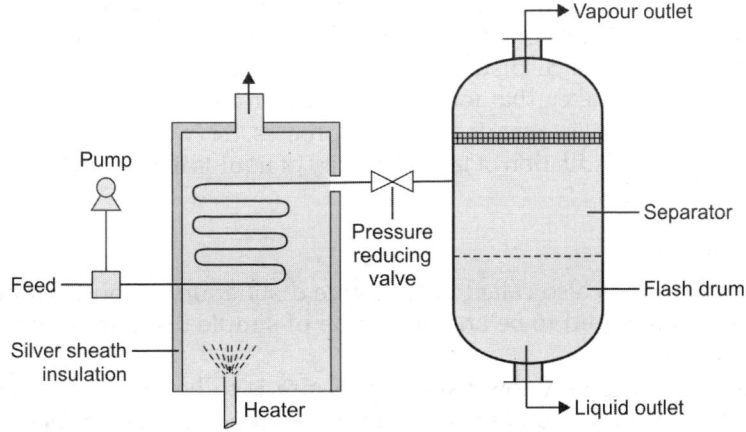

Fig. 6.9: Schematic diagram of flash distillation

Applications
- It is used for separating components that boils at widely different temperatures
- It is also used in petroleum industry for refining crude oils.

Advantages
It is useful for obtaining a multi-component system with narrow boiling point range.

Disadvantages
1. It is ineffective in separating components of comparable volatility
2. This method is not applicable when pure components are required.

Differential (Batch) Distillation
The use of distillation in batches, it means that a liquid mixture is distilled to separate it into its components before the distillation still is again charged and the process is repeated. It involves the removal of the vapour from contact with the liquid as rapidly as the vapour is formed. The solution is to evaporate only partially, because the first vapours which come off will be the richest in the more volatile component. Vapour produced later will only dilute the condensate.

The Rayleigh equation gives the final composition for a specified quantity of residual liquid if the relationship between y and x is known.

In
$$L_2/L_1 = \int_{x_1}^{x_2} 1/(y-x)$$

For each value of x between x_1 and x_2 we can look up the corresponding y value its noted and compute the integral in Rayleigh's equation $1/(y - x)$. The integral is the area under the curve between these two limits.

It is useful for the production of seasonal or low capacity and high purity chemicals. It is frequently used separating process in the pharmaceutical industry and in waste water treatment units.

Continuous Distillation
It is a regular separation technique in it a mixture is continuously fed into the process and continuously separated fractions are removed from output streams. Each of the fraction streams is taken simultaneously throughout the operation therefore a separate exit point is needed for each fraction. When there are multiple distillate fractions, a fractionating column is designed to collect distillate at different heights through a separate exit points for each distillate. From the bottom of the distillation unit the bottom fraction can be taken that may contain one or more components.

It is more often used in large scale industrial process. It is widely used in the chemical process industries for distillation of large quantity of liquids like natural gas processing, coal tar processing, etc.

Molecular Distillation
Molecular distillation is also called evaporative distillation or short path distillation or in other words it is said to be an application of simple distillation process having some modifications.

The mixtures having very low vapour pressure is to be distilled by this method which boils at very high temperatures. High vacuum must be applied in order to decrease the boiling point of such liquids.

The process is performed at an extremely low vacuum pressure. The liquid to be distillate in the distillation column is exposed to high temperature for short-term in high vacuum (around 10^{-4} mm Hg). To obtain distilled in short-time the small distance helps between the evaporator and the condenser (around 2 cm).

Compared to the simple distillation process, molecular distillation has following essential characteristics:

1. The evaporating surfaces must be close to the condensing surfaces. This is done to reduce the mean free path of the molecules. In the case of simple distillation unit for volatile liquids, the volatilization is very fast, baffles are provided to prevent entrainment, the chances of a molecule leaving the liquid and reaching the condenser are 1 in 1000. In contrast, in the molecular distillation, the close proximity of the evaporator and condenser makes the chances to 1 in 2.

2. The liquid area should be as large as possible, there is no boiling and evolution of vapour is from the surface only.

3. The process takes place under very high vacuum to minimize collisions between molecules. To ensure successful operation under high vacuum, liquids are de-gassed before distillation, there should be no leakage and pumps should be efficient.

Liquids are in the free molecular flow regime in this process, i.e. the mean free path of molecules is comparable to the size of the equipment which is defined as the average distance through which a molecule moves without coming into collision with each other.

The mean free path can be expressed:

$$\lambda = \eta \sqrt{3 / p_\rho}$$

where, λ is the mean free path, η is viscosity, p is pressure and ρ is density.

The mean free path is long for materials which are of low viscosity and density. The mean free path is low for substances that are viscous and at high pressure, but can be increased if the viscosity is decreased by elevation of temperature and pressure is reduced. So, that the substances which are non-volatile under normal temperature and pressure conditions are made volatile.

Applications

- Molecular distillation is used for purification, separation and concentration of complex and thermally sensitive molecules and also for natural products, such as vitamins and polyunsaturated fatty acids
- It is used for purification of oils in industries. It is helpful for the separation of fatty acids, steroids and triglycerides. Proteins and gums obtained as non-volatile residues
- It is used to recover to copherols from deodorizer distillate of soybean oil (DDSO) and to enrich borage oil in γ-linolenic acid (GLA)
- This is also helpful in the purification of chemicals of low vapour pressure, e.g. tricresyl phosphate, dibutyl phthalate and dimethyl phthalate.

Advantages

- This process minimizes toxicity that occurs in techniques due to the use of solvents as separating agent
- It also reduces losses due to thermal decomposition of the components
- It can be used in a continuous feed process without having break vacuum to obtain distillate.

Equipment

Molecular still can be classified into two main categories according to the method of formation of the liquid film.

1. Falling Film Molecular Still or Wiped Film Molecular Still

This is similar to wiped film evaporator or falling film evaporator. Under high vacuum the vaporization occurs which from a film of liquid. The film flows down a heated surface. The vapours travels to the condenser placed close to it and each molecule finally gets condensed individually.

Construction: The assembly of falling film molecular still is shown in Fig. 6.10. The walls are provided with arrangement of heating (jacketed) vessel having a diameter of about 1 m. Adjacent to the vessel wall wipers are located and through a rotor they are connected to a rotating head. Very close to wall of evaporating surface the condensers are arranged. The condensate is collected into a vessel. At the center of the vessel vacuum pump is connected to a large diameter pipe. Both the product and residue are collected at the bottom.

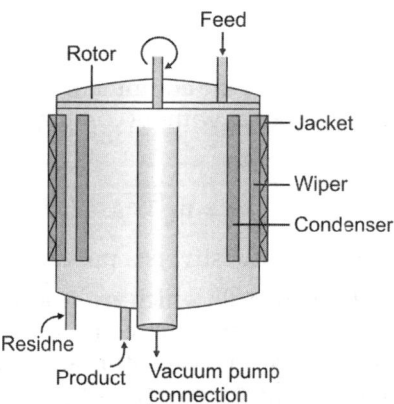

Fig. 6.10: Wiped film molecular still

Working: The vacuum is applied at the center of vessel and its wall is heated by suitable means. The liquid to be distilled enters through the feed point and wipers are allowed to rotate. The liquid flows down the walls of the vessel and spreads as a film by PTFE (poly tetra fluro ethylene) wipers that move at about 3 m/s and giving a film velocity of about 1.5 m/s. The liquid film evaporates quickly as the surface is already heated. And the vapour travels its mean free path striking the condenser. The condensate liquid is collected into a vessel and the residue (i.e. undistilled liquid which not travel to condenser) is collected at the bottom of vessel and is re-circulated.

2. Centrifugal Molecular Still

Principle: In it the liquid feed is introduced into a vessel that is rotated at very high speed in centrifugal action. The heating of liquid, vaporizes it and on the sides of vessel it form a film. The vapour gets condensed on adjacent condenser as it travels a short distance. The process condenses each molecule.

Construction: It consists of a bucket-shaped vessel having 1 to 1.5 meter diameter and rotated at high speed by a motor. To heat liquid radiant heaters are arranged externally in bucket. To the evaporating surface condensers are arranged very close and to entire vessel at the top a vacuum pump is connected. The feed is introduced in the centre of the bucket and through bottom product and residue are collected. Provisions are made for recirculation of residue (Fig. 6.11).

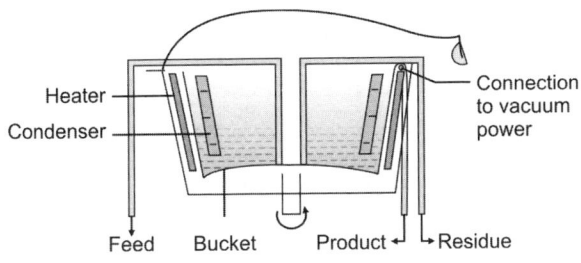

Heater
Condenser
Connection to vacuum power

Feed   Bucket   Product   Residue

Fig. 6.11: Centrifugal molecular still

Working: In it the liquid is introduced onto the centre of a bucket-shaped vessel which rotates at high speed. The liquid moves outward over the surface of the vessel and form a film due to the centrifugal action of the rotating bucket. The liquid film thus formed is heated externally by radiant heaters evaporating the liquid directly from the film. The vapour molecules strike the condenser and travels mean free path. The condensate is collected in separate vessel and the residue is re-circulated after getting collected from the bottom of vessel.

Fractional Distillation

Fractional distillation is the process in which the vaporization of liquid mixture, forms a mixture of constituents from which the component of choice can be obtained in pure form. It is also known as rectification as a part of vapour is condensed and remaining part is returned as a liquid. It is used for separating miscible liquids.

Principle: In this process separation depends upon heating the mixture repeatedly reheating the liquid and condensing the vapour and at each stage equilibrium between liquid and vapour is being set up. This can be carried out by the help of a fractionating column. This distillation is a mass transfer process, which involve a countercurrent diffusion of the components at each equilibrium stage.

It is different from simple distillation as in case of fractional distillation the vapour must passed through fractionating column where partial condensation of vapour is allowed whereas in simple distillation the vapour is directly passed through condenser. In simple distillation, condensate is collected from receiver whereas in fractional distillation condensation takes place in the fractionating column so part of the condensing vapour goes back into the still.

Applications

- Fractional distillation is used to separate miscible volatile liquids having close boiling points, e.g. acetone-water, chloroform-benzene
- It is not used to separate miscible liquids which form azeotropic mixtures.

Equipment for Fractional Distillation

In a laboratory assembly for fractional distillation it consist of bunsen burner, round-bottomed flask, condenser and the single-purpose fractionating column. The fractionating column is inserted between the still and the condenser. Bunsen burner is used as source to supply heat at the bottom of the column. The fractionating column provides large surface area for sufficient flow of liquid. At the top of column a condenser is connected. The broken lines present inside the column represent the contacting devices (Fig. 6.12).

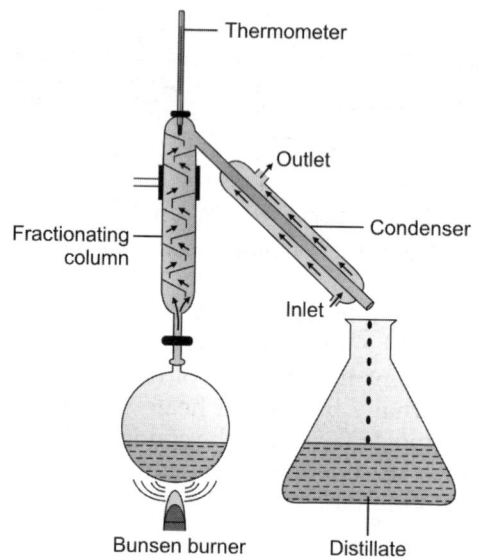

Fig. 6.12: Laboratory scale fractional distillation apparatus

Working

The apparatus in this diagram represents a batch apparatus as opposed to a continuous apparatus. The fractionating column is fitted into the top and the mixture is put into the round bottomed flask along with a few anti-bumping granules. On the still pot the heat source is set-up at the bottom. A temperature gradient is formed in the column as there is increase in the distance from the stillpot. The column is found to be coolest at the top and hottest at the bottom. Some of the vapour condenses and revaporizes along the temperature gradient as the mixed vapour ascends the temperature gradient. Each time the vapour condenses and vaporizes the composition of the more volatile component in the vapour increases. Eventually, the vapour is composed solely of the more volatile component (or an azeotrope) and this distills the vapour along the length of the column. Inside the column the vapour condenses on the glass platforms known as trays and runs back down refluxing distillate into the liquid below. Hottest tray is kept at the bottom and the coolest is at the top. The vapour and liquid on each tray are at equilibrium at the steady state conditions. The most volatile component exits from the mixture as gas at the top of the column. At the top of the column, the vapour goes to the condenser where it cools down until it liquefies. The separation is more effective to get pure fractions if the number tray is more (at specific heat, flow, etc.). The first condensate will be close to the azeotropic composition and the condensate becomes gradually richer in water when most of the ethanol has been removed. This process continues till the entire ethanol boils out of the mixture. This point can be known by the sharp rise in temperature. In terms of the amount of heating and time required to get fractionation the efficiency of the process can be improved by insulating from outside of the column by using of wool, aluminium foil or preferably a vacuum jacket.

Several types of condensers are commonly found in laboratory distillation. The Liebig condenser is the simplest (and relatively least expensive) form of condenser having a straight tube within a water jacket. The Graham condenser is a spiral tube within a water jacket and the Allihn condenser has a series of large and small constrictions on the inside tube, each increasing the surface area upon which the vapour constituents may condense.

Large Scale Assembly for Fractional Distillation

It is the most common separation technology widely used and is operated at a continuous steady state in petroleum refineries, chemical plants, natural gas processing, cryogenic air separation plants, etc. Always new feed is being added to the distillation column and products are being removed. The amount of feed being added and the amount of product being removed are normally equal and this is known as continuous, steady-state fractional distillation.

In large scale, industrial distillation process a distillation columns also known as "fractionation towers" a vertical cylindrical having diameters between 65 centimeters to 6 meters and heights from 6 meters to 60 meters or more have been used. This cylindrical towers have outlets for liquids at various intervals up the column which is used for the exit of different fractions or products having different boiling points, e.g.

This process is used in oil refineries to separate crude oil into useful substances (or fractions) that are having different hydrocarbons of different boiling points (Fig. 6.13).

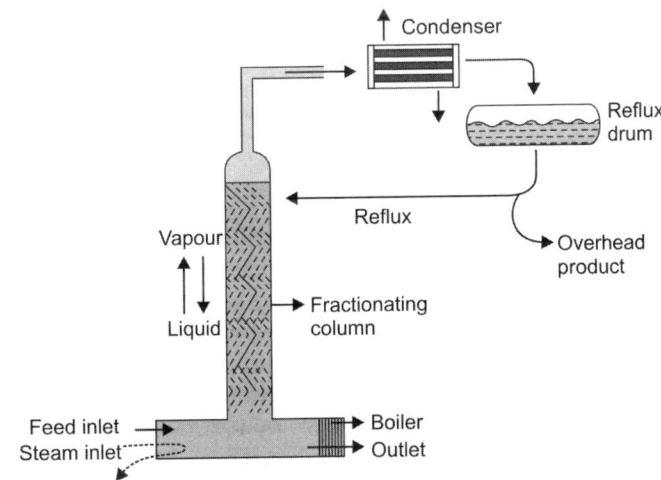

Fig. 6.13: Schemmatic diagram of large scale fractional distillation

For the complete separation of products the large-scale industrial towers use reflux. The reflux refers to the portion which is obtained of condensed overhead liquid product from a fractionation tower or distillation unit and is goes to the upper part of the tower as shown in the diagram.

After entered into the tower, the reflux liquid flowing downwards and provides the cooling effect required to condense the vapours flowing upwards. By this it is increasing the efficiency of the distillation tower.

For a given number of theoretical plates, the more reflux is provided, better is the tower's separation of lower boiling materials from higher boiling materials.

Alternatively, the fewer theoretical plates are required and more reflux is provided for a given desired separation.

Applications

- Separation of various fractions of crude oil is performed by fractional distillation
- It is also used in producing liquid oxygen, liquid nitrogen, and highly concentrated argon and also in air separation
- Distillation of chlorosilanes enables the production of high-purity silicon which is used as a semiconductor.

Efficiency of the Fractional Distillation

Many factors denote the efficiency of fractional distillation:

Length of the fractionating column: For efficient separation, a dynamic equilibrium must establish. A maximum degree of separation of component is achieved in longer column.

Reflux ratio: During the same interval of time the ratio of the amount of liquid returning through the column to the amount collected into the receiver is known as reflux ratio. Reflux ratio should be high for efficient separation and is controlled by the help of a suitable still.

Heat input: Sufficient heat must be provided throughout the column. The heat is provided in controlled manner. It is too low, the packing is insufficiently wetted. If it is too high, the velocity of the liquid may be too great to attain equilibrium. The size of the heat input must be adjusted so that liquid passes over a rate of one drop for every 2–3 seconds.

Column temperature: The heat loss through the column must be prevented by insulation. The column is surrounded by a heating jacket, such as asbestos cord and silver vacuum jacket.

Fractionating Columns

Most commercial operations require a relatively complete separation between two components. This can be achieved in a column which is capable of producing from a single feed a distillate product containing only a small amount of the less-volatile component and a bottom product containing a very small amount of the more volatile component. A stripping column produces a bottom product which is relatively free from the more volatile component, and a rectifying column produces a product which is relatively free from the less volatile component. The complete fractionating column includes a rectifying section above the feed plate and a stripping section below the feed plate. The feed enters the fractionating column on the feed plate which is top plate of the stripping section. The total liquid entering the top plate of the stripping section is composed of the feed liquid and liquid overflowing from the rectifying section above the feed plate. The purpose of the stripping section is to remove the more volatile component from the total liquid entering the stripping section in order to produce a bottom product nearly free of the more volatile product. The total vapour entering the bottom plate of the rectifying section is composed of the feed vapour and vapour rising from the stripping section below the feed plate. The purpose of the rectifying section is to remove the less volatile component from the total vapour entering the rectifying section in order to produce a distillate product nearly free of the less volatile product.

Design and Control of Fractionating Columns

Design of a fractionating column includes the number of actual plates, the dimension of column, its components including risers, downspouts, spacing of plates, packing and its support.

The Number of Actual Plates

The overall plate efficiency is defined as the number of equilibrium stages required for a given separation divided by the number of actual plates required.

Bubble Caps

A bubble cap assembly consists of a chimney or riser, the cap which is mounted over the riser and some means of holding the cap in place. The spacing of the caps on a plate should be such as to give ample turbulence to the liquid around the caps but not so close as to produce spouting or jetting between the caps. The design of the cap is such that the area of the chimney is equal to the area of the annular space between the cap and the chimney. These areas are also approximately equal to the area of the slots.

A bubble cap plate is a plate pierced with a number of holes into which are fitted risers or chimneys through which vapours from the plate below may pass. Each of the risers is covered by a bell-shaped cap which is fastened to the risers by means of a spider or any other mounting. The caps are mounted to provide sufficient space between the riser and the cap to allow passage of vapours. The lower edge of the bubble cap may be serrated, or the skirt of the cap may be pierced with a number of slots. In operation, vapour rises through the chimney and is directed downwards by the cap, discharging as small bubbles from the slots or notches at the bottom of the cap beneath the liquid. Liquid is fed to the plate and passes across it and down through the downspout to the plate below, while the vapours pass upward through the plate, mixing intimately with the liquid on the plate because of the dispersion produced by the slots in the bubble caps. The vapours then separate at the liquid surface and pass to the plate above. Thus, the countercurrent flow of liquid passing downward and vapour passing upward through the column is obtained.

Sieve plates are those in which the bubble cap assembly is replaced by small holes in the plate. The construction of downspouts and weirs is identical to that used in the bubble cap columns.

The packed tower consists of a vertical shell which is filled with suitable packing material. The liquid flows over the surface of packing in thin films, thereby presenting a large liquid surface in contact with ascending gases. The packing is supported on a suitable grid. The liquid is introduced at the top of the packing by means of a distributing plate (a perforated plate) and the vapour is introduced beneath the grid which supports the packing. The packed towers are advantageous in terms of multiple-contact and countercurrent flow but the plate type towers provide efficiency of contacting.

Risers or Chimneys

If the plate is cast the risers may be cast as a part of the plate. Otherwise, they may be welded or brazed to the plate, or they may be rolled, screwed, or clamped into place.

Downspouts

They are circular conduits through which liquid passes from a plate to the plate below, or chord-shaped where the raised edge of the downspouts serves as a weir.

Azeotropic Distillation

Azeotropic mixture cannot be separated by fractional distillation because at any time either vapour or liquid in still has mixture of components. Therefore, azeotropic distillation is designed to separate such constant boiling mixture by addition of external substance called entrainer which affects the volatility of one of the azeotropic more than the other. When a new substance is added to an azeotropic mixture, a binary mixture broken and a ternary azeotrope result. The distillation of mixture is called azeotropic distillation.

For example, benzene to water/ethanol azeotrope, cyclohexane to water/ethanol azeotrope. The relative volatility of the liquid mixture can be changed by the addition of a substance. When benzene was added to the water/ethanol mixture a ternary azeotrope is formed which increase the volatility of water. Water is distilled at 65.85° cleaving benzene and alcohol. This binary mixture boils at 68.5°C and benzene gets distilled leaving pure ethanol.

MATHEMATICAL PROBLEMS

1. You have a solution of 5.54 g of sugar (sucrose, $C_{12}H_{22}O_{11}$) in 90.0 g of water.
   a. Calculate the moles of sugar and water present in solution. (H = 1, C = 12, O = 16)
   b. What will be the mole fraction of the water in the solution.
   c. Calculate the vapour pressure of the solution at 100°C (saturated vapour pressure of water at this temperature is 101325 Pa).

Solution:

a. Mole of sugar = wt. of sugar taken/molecular wt. of sugar

$\qquad$ = 5.54/342

$\qquad$ = 0.0161 moles

$\quad$ Mole of water = 90.0/18

$\qquad$ = 5 moles

b. Mole fraction water in solution = moles of water/(moles of sugar + moles of water)

$\qquad$ = 5/5.016

$\qquad$ = 0.997

c. Vapour pressure of the solution = vapour pressure of sugar + vapour pressure of water

$\quad$ Vapour pressure of sugar = vp of pure sugar × mole fraction of sugar

2. A mixture containing 0.5 mole fraction of benzene and 0.5 mole fraction of toluene at 95.25°C. What is the actual vapour pressure of benzene and toluene in the liquid mixture? Vapour pressure of benzene and toluene at this temperature is 1180 mmHg and 481 mm Hg respectively.

Solution:

Vapour pressure of the mixture (P) = vapour pressure of toluene (P_A) + vapour pressure of benzene (P_B)

Vapour pressure of toluene (P_A) = 481 × 0.5 = 240.5 mm Hg

Vapour pressure of benzene (P_B) = 1180 × 0.5 = 295 mm Hg

3. Turpentine oil (molecular weight = 136) and water mixture is to distilled at atmospheric pressure. The boiling point of the mixture is 95.6°C. The vapour pressure of pure water at this temperature is 645 mm Hg. Find the ratio of the oil in the distillate. (Boiling point of turpentine oil is 160°C).

Solution:

Weight ratio of distillate $= m_A/m_B = po_A \, M_A/po_B \, M_B$

$$= \text{Water/oil} = 18 \times 645/136 \times 113$$

$$= 1/1.32$$

VERY SHORT QUESTIONS

1. Define the process of distillation. How it differ from extraction?

2. Describe Raoult's law and its significance.

3. Discuss the deviation from Raoult's law with suitable example.

4. Define azeotropic mixtures with suitable examples.

5. Define volatility and relative volatility.

6. Discuss phase rule in detail with its significance.

SHORT QUESTIONS

1. Discuss the principle of separation of binary mixture of immiscible liquids.

2. What is the difference between simple distillation and steam distillation?

3. Explain with suitable diagram the process of flash distillation carried out in the laboratory.

4. Explain the principle, design and working of rectification.

5. What is a theoretical plate in fractionating column?

6. Write note on packed column used in fractional distillation.

7. Discuss the efficiency of fractionating columns.

LONG QUESTIONS

1. What is HETP? How it is calculated?

2. Derive equations for overall heat and material balances for a continuous fractionating column.

3. Describe the design and working of bubble cap rectifying column.

4. Discuss the principle and equipment in detail of molecular distillation. What are the applications of molecular distillation in industry?

5. Explain the process of steam distillation with the help of suitable diagram. Discuss the design and working of it for laboratory purpose.

6. Define rectification. What are the factors which affect the efficiency of rectification?

7. Write note on distillation under reduced pressure.

MULTIPLE CHOICE QUESTIONS

1. .... is the process of heating a liquid mixture to form vapours' and then cooling them to get pure component.
   a. Crystallisation
   b. Distillation
   c. Chromatography
   d. Sublimation

2. The pieces of porcelain are put in the distillation flask to avoid:
   a. Overheating
   b. Uniform boiling
   c. Bumping of the solution
   d. None of the mentioned options

3. The distilled is collected in:
   a. Reciever
   b. Adapter
   c. Condenser
   d. Round bottom flask

4. Distillation process is used for the liquids that have:
   a. Sufficient difference in their boiling point
   b. Sufficient difference in their melting point
   c. Sufficient difference in their solubility
   d. None of the mentioned

5. The residue that remains left in the round bottom flask are:
   a. Volatile
   b. Non-volatile
   c. Both a and b
   d. None of above

6. .... azeotropes are formed by adding the entrainer:
   a. Low boiling
   b. High boiling
   c. No
   d. None of above

7. The solvent is use for increasing the relative volatility in:
   a. Multi-component distillation
   b. Reactive distillation
   c. Azeotropic distillation
   d. Extractive distillation

8. Use of heat in the distillation is to separate the distillate from the entrainer.
   a. True
   b. False

9. Choose the azeotropic mixture:
   a. Air-water
   b. Acetic acid-water
   c. Acetic acid-alcohol
   d. Air-alcohol

10. Batch distillation also known as:
    a. Flash distillation
    b. Rayleigh's criteria
    c. Thompson distillation
    d. Crane distillation

11. .... is also called flash distillation.
    a. Final distillation
    b. Equilibrium distillation
    c. Growth distillation
    d. Full distillation

12. **The suitable method for a substance to decompose if heated to its boiling point is:**
    a. Simple distillation
    b. Fractional distillation
    c. Vacuum distillation
    d. Crystallization

13. **Higher the column in fractionating column of fractional distillation:**
    a. The temperature becomes lower
    b. The temperature becomes higher
    c. Minimum absorption is carried out
    d. Risks of sublimation exists

14. **The substance boils at .... in vacuum distillation.**
    a. Its exact temperature
    b. Temperature slightly above its boiling point
    c. A temperature below its boiling point
    d. Under high pressures

15. **After distillation distillate formed is:**
    a. A diluted solution
    b. May contain impurities
    c. A condensed solution
    d. A concentrated solution

16. **To produce .... crude oil can be fractionally distilled.**
    a. Diesel
    b. Petrol
    c. Paraffin
    d. All of these

17. **Distillation process is performed at an extremely low vacuum pressure, 0.01 torr or below is:**
    a. Simple distillation
    b. Molecular distillation
    c. Flash distillation
    d. Fraction distillation

18. **Efficiency of the fractional distillation depends upon:**
    a. Column temperature
    b. Heat input
    c. Reflux ratio
    d. All of above

Drying

Yasmin Sultana and Md. Thasleem

Drying is defined as the removal of small amounts of water or any other liquid from a material by the application of heat.

OBJECTIVES

Drying is commonly utilized in the last stage of the process and has considerable importance. Drying means complete dryness or a condition known as air dry. The liquid can be organic, such as chloroform, ethanol and isopropanol. Drying is also applied for removal of small quantities of water or liquid from gases, as in case of drying of gases. The liquid may be removed from the solids mechanically by a filter press or centrifuge or as vapours by application of heat. Mechanical methods of removal of liquids is less expensive than thermal methods therefore, much amount of liquids is removed mechanically before subjecting the material to thermal drying.

Drying and evaporation are distinguished by the relative quantities of liquid removed from the solid. In evaporation the product obtained is either concentrated solution or suspension or wet slurry. In drying dry solid is the product. In evaporation, water is removed at its boiling point, but in drying, vapour is removed at a temperature below its boiling point.

Drying is possible when the environment is not saturated with the water vapour. Therefore, humidity in the environment is an important determinant for drying of the solids.

APPLICATIONS

Drying step is essential after certain operations, such as crystallization and filtration. And also as a prerequisite for operations like size reduction. If moisture is present, size reduction of drugs is difficult. Drying reduces the moisture content.

Preparation of bulk drugs: Drying is the last stage in the processing of bulk drugs. Few examples are, powdered extracts, spray dried lactose and dried aluminum hydroxide.

Preservation of drug products: Drying is necessary in order to avoid deterioration of many products; to prevent chemical decomposition of crude drugs of animal and vegetable origin; and microbial degradation of blood products.

Improved characteristic: Drying produces materials of uniform spherical shape with free flowing and enhanced solubility characteristics. Granules are dried to improve compression properties which are essential for the production of tablets and capsules. Drying is used to modify characteristics of viscous and sticky materials like malt extract and oleo resin to make them free flowing.

Improved Handling

Drying is used to reduce weight of material which cuts down cost of transportation.

THEORY OF DRYING

In a wet solid mass, water may be present as bound water and unbound water.

Bound water (moisture) is the minimum water held up by the material which exerts an equilibrium vapour pressure less than that of pure water at the same temperature.

Unbound water (moisture) is the amount of water (moisture) held by the material which exerts an equilibrium vapour pressure that is equal to that of pure water at the same temperature.

During drying, though water is lost, but the resulting solid is not completely free from water molecules. At that stage it is known as air-dry. Unbound water is easily removable at the defined environmental conditions. When water is removed completely, the material is said to be 'bone-dry'.

Unbound water is present largely in the voids of the solid. Thus, in a non-hygroscopic material, all the liquid exists as unbound water. In a hygroscopic material, the unbound moisture is the liquid in excess of the equilibrium moisture content, corresponding to saturation humidity. Substances containing bound water are often called *hygroscopic substances*. The distinction between bound and unbound water depends on the material itself.

Heat must be transferred to the material to be dried in order to supply the latent heat required for vapourisation of the moisture. Water diffuses though the material to the surface and subsequently evaporates into the air steam. Thus drying involves both heat transfer and mass transfer operations simultaneously.

MECHANISM OF DRYING PROCESS

Drying involves simultaneous heat transfer and mass transfer process. Transfer of heat takes place from the heating medium to the solid material. Mass transfer involves the transfer of moisture to the surface of the solids and subsequently vapourisaton from the surface into surroundings. The movement of moisture is proposed by few theories: Diffusion theory, capillary theory, pressure gradient theory, gravity flow theory, vapourisation and condensation mechanisms. In diffusion theory, the rate of flow of water is proportional to moisture gradient. According to this theory, water diffuses through the solid to the surface and subsequently evaporates into the surroundings. Due to limitations in predicting the drying rate over a range of moisture gradients, this theory is not much applicable. Capillary theory is applicable to porous granular solids. Porous material contains a network of inter-connected pores and channels, and at the surface, the cross-section of these capillaries forms various sizes of pores. As the drying starts, a meniscus is formed in the capillary and exerts a force. This is the driving forces for the movement of water though pores towards the surface. Capillary theory holds good only for free water in the bed. This type of movement of liquid takes place in granules pores as well as in the spaces between the granules (void spaces). As the pore diameter is considerably smaller inside a granule than the surrounding granules, liquid surrounding the granules can be removed initially. Then liquid inside a granule is vapourised. Pressure gradient theory is applicable to drying of solids by the application of radiation. Radiation is a source for generating internal heat. The radiation interacts with the polarised molecules and ions of the material. This field aligns the molecules in order, which are otherwise randomly oriented. When the field is reversed, the molecules return to the original orientation. In this process, it gives up random kinetic energy (or heat) to the inside surface of the solids itself. Therefore, liquid inside the solids is vapourised. As a result, vapour pressure gradient is developed which is the driving force for the movement of vapour to the surface. This type of drying mechanism is applicable to radiation drying, provided such rays penetrate deep inside the solid mass.

RATE OF DRYING CURVE

Consider drying of sand in an insulated tray which is an example of porous, insoluble material. The hot air passing over the surface of sand serves as the drying medium. The hot drying medium supplies all the heat required for vapourisation of water and the heating of the solid. If the drying medium passes over the slab of solid at a sufficient velocity so that its temperature, velocity and humidity are unaffected by the transfer of water vapour from the solid slab to the drying medium, data are obtained which indicates the water content of the slab (expressed as pounds of water per pound of water-free solid) as a function of drying rate (expressed as pounds of water per hour per pound of water-free solid) (Fig. 7.1). Such a curve is a typical rate curve which may be divided into several distinct periods as the moisture content of the slab is reduced from the high initial value to the final value, as follows:

Period I_0: An initial phase of short duration during which the drying rate may increase or decrease rapidly from an initial value.

Period I: An early stage of drying during which the drying rate remains constant.

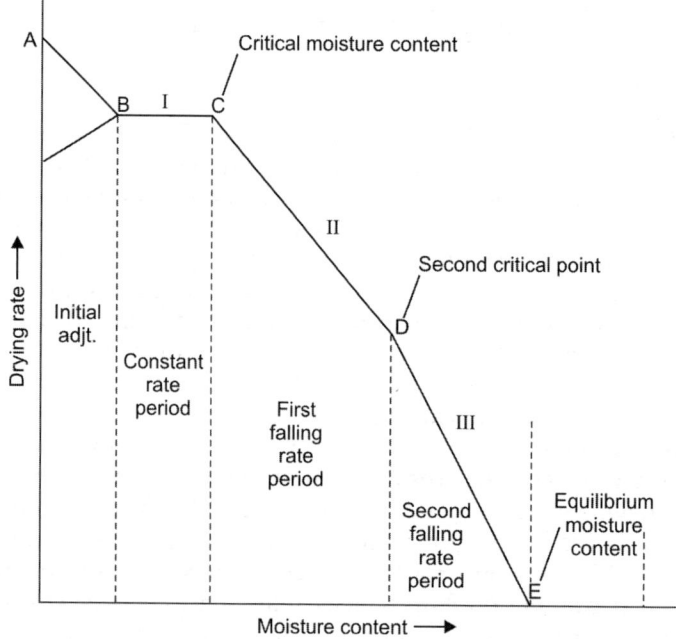

Fig. 7.1: Typical rate curve

Period II: A period of drying during which the drying rate decreases, more or less linearly with the continued decrease in the water content of solid.

Period III: A stage of drying immediately following period II, during which the drying rate decreases more or less linearly with decreasing water content.

On prolonged drying under constant conditions, the rate at which the slab of solid is dried, becomes zero. The limit to which the water content can be reduced by drying for an infinite length of time is known as the equilibrium moisture content. The equilibrium moisture content X^* is the limit to which a given material can be dried by means of a drying medium of given temperature and humidity. It depends on the nature of the solid material, the temperature of the drying medium, and the partial pressure of the water vapour in the drying medium. A nonporous highly insoluble material may have equilibrium moisture content of practically zero, whereas some organic materials, such as soap, leather and wood have equilibrium moisture contents which may vary over wide ranges, depending upon temperature and humidity of the drying medium. The water which makes up the equilibrium moisture content of a given solid may be adsorbed in the solid, it may be held by capillary forces in the pores of the solid, or it may be in chemical combination with the solid. The difference between the total moisture content X and the equilibrium moisture content X^* is known as free moisture content, F and is expressed as pounds of water per pound of dry solid.

$$F = X - X^*$$

When the slab is initially cold, i.e. below the adiabatic saturation temperature of the drying medium, then the heat is transferred to the relatively cold wet surface of the slab from the relatively hot drying medium. It raises the temperature of the water in the slab to the temperature at which evaporation takes place and supplies the latent heat of vapourisation. The driving potential for the evaporation of water from the surface of slab into the drying medium is the difference in the vapour pressure of the surface of slab and the partial pressure of the water vapour in the drying medium. As this process continues, with the increase in the surface temperature, there is an increase in the evaporation rate and a corresponding decrease in the rate at which heat is transferred to the slab. After a short period of time, the rate of heat transfer becomes equal to the heat required for evaporation, and rate of evaporation attained a constant value at approximately the wet-bulb temperature.

When the slab is initially hotter than the wet bulb temperature of the drying medium, the latent heat requirement is greater than that transferred to the slab and the drying rate decreases to the steady condition. When the initial temperature of the slab is at the adiabatic saturation temperature of the drying medium, no initial varying period is observed and the drying started at the constant drying rate.

Period I the constant drying rate period, begins at the free moisture content F_1 and ends at the critical moisture content F_2, is characterised by the uniform rate of drying and a constant surface and interior temperature of the slab. It is a steady-state period. This period continues as long as water is supplied to the surface of slab as fast as evaporation takes place. When the rate at which water is supplied to the surface of the slab becomes less than the rate at which evaporation can occur, the rate of drying decreases and period I of constant rate drying terminates.

Period II, the first falling rate period starts at the free moisture content F_2 and ends at F_3. It is characterised by a decreasing rate of evaporation which results from decrease in the evaporation surface. The heat supplied causes an increase in the temperature at the decreased zone of evaporation. As drying proceeds the fraction of wetted surface decreases to zero. This is the time when all evaporation becomes subsurface and period II terminates.

Period III, the second falling rate period starts when the capillary flow to the surface has ceased, and continues under prolonged time to the point when the stock is at its equilibrium moisture content, X^*. In this period, evaporation takes place below the surface layers and the area from which evaporation takes place decreases continuously. There is a necessity for heat of evaporation to penetrate increasing thickness of partially dried material.

EQUILIBRIUM RELATIONSHIPS AND EMC

Exposure to air at a definite temperature and humidity will cause a material to lose or gain moisture until an equilibrium moisture content is attained. The values of EMC depends upon the temperature and humidity of the air and on the properties of the material being dried. EMC values are low with non-porous solids, but higher and variable with fibrous or colloidal organic substances. Equilibrium moisture content (EMC) is the amount of water present in the solid which exerts a vapour pressure equal to the vapour pressure of the atmosphere surrounding it.

The moisture (content) which is more difficult to remove in practice is the equilibrium moisture content. This moisture content is retained by the solid under steady state conditions. This water (or liquid) does not vapourise or produce vapour pressure. Measurement of EMC.

Equilibrium moisture content can be represented as curves in which for a particular temperature, moisture content is plotted against relative humidity. For determination of EMC, solids to be dried were placed in a petridish and it was kept in oven. Oven temperature is regulated and after fixed intervals of time, petridish removed from oven, lid was kept open for a few seconds and its weight was taken. This procedure was repeated till three consecutive equal weights were obtained. Moisture content was determined from the formula:

Moisture content at given time = Weight of initial sample – weight of sample at given time/weight of initial sample.

Then, moisture content values were plotted against time. A graph is obtained (Fig. 7.2), the horizontal portion in the curve is extrapolated to Y-axis to obtain EMC value at that temperature for the material.

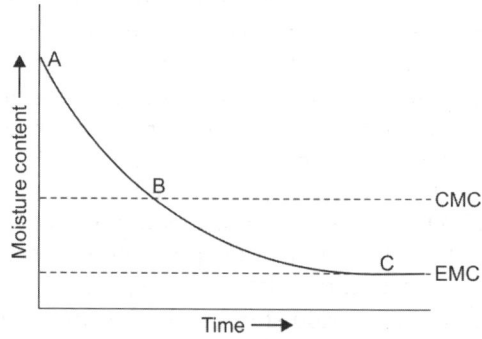

CMC: Critical moisture content
EMC: Equilibrium moisture content

Fig. 7.2: Drying curve

Application of EMC: The EMC curve allows the selection of the experimental conditions to be used for drying the product. When the moisture content reaches the level of the EMC under the exposed conditions, drying should be discontinued. Since over-dried solid quickly regain the moisture from the ambient conditions, therefore over drying should be avoided.

If the moisture content is to be reduced, the relative humidity of the ambient air must be reduced as a first step. This can be done mechanically on a large scale using an air-conditioning system. On a small-scale, desiccators are employed. Some materials, such as tablet granules, have superior compaction properties with a small amount (1–2%) of residual moisture content.

Factors affecting EMC: EMC values depends on the *nature of material and properties of air.* Non-porous insoluble solids have an EMC of practically zero, e.g. talc. The EMC values are high and variable for fibrous or colloidal organic substances.

The EMC values are much higher for porous solids as the water may be held in fine capillaries that have no access to the surface. EMC of all materials is zero for air of zero humidity and as the temperature of air increases, the EMC of solid decreases.

EMC of solids is a constant for a given temperature and humidity of air. If the equilibrium curves are continued up to 100% RH, the moisture content so obtained (EMC with saturated air) is the least moisture at which the material can exert a vapour pressure as high as that exerted by liquid water at the same temperature.

Free moisture content (FMC): Free moisture content (FMC) is the amount of water which is free to evaporate from the solid surface.

Under the conditions of saturation humidity (100% RH), the EMC is the minimum moisture content. Under these conditions the water must be bound water which is minimum at that temperature. The remaining is unbound for which the FMC for a given condition can be written as:

Free moisture content (FMC) = total water content – equilibrium moisture content (EMC)

The distinction between free and equilibrium moisture depends on the drying conditions.

Rate Relationships

Rate relationship can be studied by considering simple model, which mimic the condition as of a dryer. Based on this model, the wet slab need to be dried is properly positioned on a tray endowed with bottom and side insulation. The solid is subjected to uniform drying air conditions by keeping constant air velocity, temperature, pressure and humidity. The water content present in the superficial area gets imbibed to the nearer stagnant air film followed by the fast moving stream of air. The slab weighing is performed on periodic manner to estimate the moisture loss from the relative weight difference of adjacent periods. The remaining moisture of solid is regarded as wet weight or dry weight. This is expressed by calculation as following:

$$\% \text{ Loss on drying (LOD)} = \frac{\text{Mass of water in sample (kg)}}{\text{Total mass of wet sample (kg)}} \times 100$$

$$\% \text{ Moisture content (MC)} = \frac{\text{Mass of water in sample (kg)}}{\text{Total mass of dry sample (kg)}} \times 100$$

$$\text{Drying rate} = \frac{\text{Weight of water in sample (kg)}}{\text{Time (h)} \times \text{weight of the dry solid (kg)}} \times 100$$

EQUIPMENT

Tray Dryer

Principle: In tray dryer, there is continuous circulation of hot air. Forced convection heating takes place to remove moisture from the solids which are placed in trays.

Construction: It is a cabinet with a heater at the bottom to assist convection and a fan for forced convection. The construction of a tray dryer is shown in Fig. 7.3. It consists of a rectangular chamber with insulated walls. Trays are placed in the heating chamber. The number of tray increase with the size of the dryer. Each tray is rectangular or square in shape and about 1.2 to 2.4 meters square in area. The distance between the bottom of upper tray and (upper) surface of the material loaded in the subsequent tray must be 40.0 millimeters.

Alternately, the trays can be placed in trucks on wheels that are rolled into and out of chamber. Two such trucks can be arranged inside dryer. There is a fan for circulating air over the trays in the dryer. Electrically heated elements are provided inside the dryer to heat the air. In the corner of the chamber, direction vanes are placed to direct air flow path.

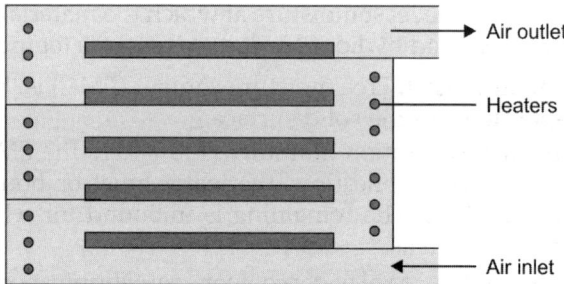

Fig. 7.3: Compartment dryer (tray dryer)

Working: Heaters are placed in such a way that the air is re-heated before passing over each shelf so, that the air temperature is minimised. As the air passes over each shelf, it gives certain amount of heat as latent heat of vapourisation. The hot air is circulated by means of fans, turbulent flow lowers the partial vapour pressure in the atmosphere and also reduces the thickness of the air boundary layer. As water evaporates from the surface, the water diffuses from the interior of the solid by capillary action. The re-heating method reduces the air temperature and amount of air which is needed to carry the same moisture level. In addition, the air outlet is connected to the inlet so that air is re-circulated. Thus, the equipment provides economy of heat. Moist air is discharged through outlet. Thus constant temperature and uniform air flow over the material can be maintained for achieving uniform drying.

In case of wet granules (as in tablets and capsules) drying is continued until the desired moisture content is obtained. At the end of drying, trays (trucks) are pulled out of the chamber and taken to a tray dumping station.

Uses: The tray drier is a very versatile drier and its applications include drying of crude drugs, chemicals, powders, tablet granules, or items of equipment. Sticky materials, plastic substances, granular mass or crystal line materials, precipitates and pastes can be dried in a tray dryer. Crude drugs, chemicals, powders, tablet granules or parts of equipment are dried.

Advantages

- In tray dryer, there are no losses during handling of materials (loading and unloading)
- Batch wise operation is used extensively in the manufacture of pharmaceutical due to the reason that every batch in a tray dryer is dried separately and unlike chemical industry, each batch would be quite smaller in size with approximately 250 kg or less in each batch.

Disadvantages: Tray dryer is a time consuming process requiring relatively large manpower. This contributes to increase in cost.

Variants: The drying process of tray dryer is executed under vacuum conditions even with indirect heating. This type of special vacuum dryer is especially useful for drying heat sensitive materials like vitamins.

Tunnel dryer: In this type, trucks are loaded with wet material at one end of the tunnel. The tunnel comprised of a number of units each of which is electro-statically controlled. The solids get dried and the product is discharged at the other end of the tunnel.

Drum Dryer or Roller Dryer (or Film Drum Dryer)

Principle: In a drum drier, the fluid is spread in a thin film upon the outer surface of a heated, rotating drum. As the drum rotates the fluid get dried by the evaporation of the solvent. The dried product is removed from the drum as the drum moves past a knife or scraper.

Construction: The construction of a drum dryer is shown in Fig. 7.4. It consists of a horizontally mounted hollow steel drum with smoothly polished external surface. Feed pan is placed below the drum in such a way that the drum dips partially into the feed. A spreader is placed on one side of drum and on the other side a doctor's knife is placed to scrap the dried material. A conveyor is placed to collect the material.

Working: Steam is passed through the drum. The drum metal has high heat transfer coefficient. Drying capacity of dryer is directly proportional to the surface area of the drum. Conduction is used to transfer heat to the material. At the same time drum is

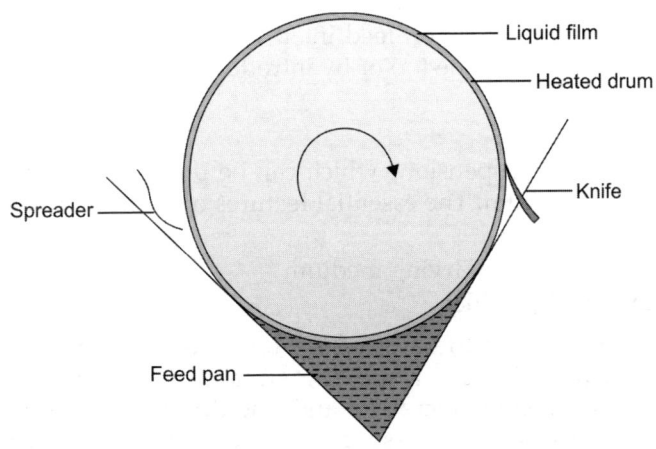

Fig. 7.4: Drum dryer

rotated at a rate of 1–10 revolutions per minute. As the heated drum rotates, the liquid material present in the feed pan adheres as a thin layer to the external surface of drum. Complete drying of the material is obtained during its passage in slightly less than one rotation (i.e. from one side to another side of the drum). Dried material is scrapped by the doctor's knife and stored into a storage bin. The duration of contact of the material with hot metal is 6 to 15 seconds only. Hence, processing conditions, such as film thickness, steam temperature are closely controlled. The efficiency of drying product may be controlled by the temperature and speed of the drums. As drying takes place in thin films, products are removed as a flake, which enhances sales appeal of the material. For materials which do not adhere to the heated surface, spraying or splashing as a method of feeding is used.

Uses: This type of drier is suitable for handling heat sensitive materials as the material is exposed to the heated zone for relatively short periods. Drum dryer is used for drying solutions, slurries, suspensions, etc. the products dried are milk product, starch products, ferrous salts, suspensions of zinc oxide, suspension of kaolin yeast pigments, malt extracts, antibiotics, glandular extracts, insecticides, DDT, calcium and barium carbonates.

Advantages

- In drum dryer, drying time is only a few seconds. Therefore heat sensitive, materials can be dried
- Drum dryer occupies less space, as it is compact when compared to spray dryer
- As a thin film of liquid is formed on the large heating surface, rates of heat transfer and mass transfer are high.

Disadvantages

- Drum dryer has a high maintenance cost than spray dryer
- It requires skilled operators to control feed rate, film thickness, speed of rotation and temperature
- Solutions of salts with less solubility are not dried by this method.

Variants: A vacuum drum dryer encloses both drum and feed line in a vacuum chamber to facilities drying of heat sensitive materials. It is suitable for drying of drugs susceptible to oxidation and to recover solvents.

In a large scale, instead of one drum, two drums are set in parallels, rotating in opposite directions with a common feed inlet. The feed can be introduced onto the drum either by spraying it on the top or by introducing from the bottom.

SPRAY DRYER

Principle: Solutions and suspensions which can be pumped may be sprayed into a stream of the drying medium. The essential features of a spray drier are:
- Means of fluid dispersion
- Contact between spray and drying medium
- Recovery of the dried product.

In spray dryer, the liquid to be dried is atomized in the form of fine droplets which are thrown radially into a moving stream of hot gas. Immediately, the temperature of the droplets is increased and fine droplets get dried in the form of spherical particles. This process takes a few a seconds before the droplets reach the wall of the dryer.

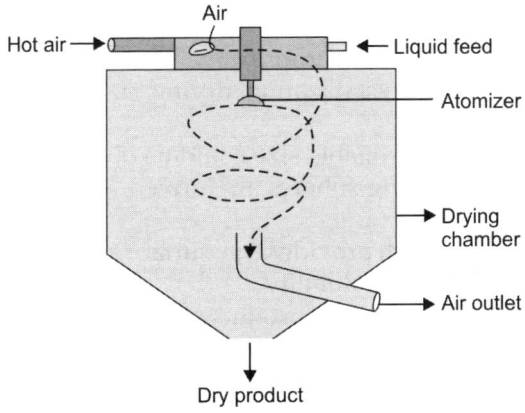

Fig. 7.5: Spray dryer

Construction: The construction of a spray dryer is shown in Fig. 7.5. It consists of a large cylindrical drying chamber and a short conical bottom, an inlet for hot air is placed at the top. The spray disk atomizer is about 300 millimeters in diameter and rotates at a speed of 3,000 to 50,000 revolutions per minute. The bottom of the dryer is connected to a cyclone separator.

Direct air heater is replaced by an indirect steam heater to ensure that the product is free from contamination. Air filters may also be used. Centrifugal disk nozzles or pressure nozzles are used to disperse or spray the fluid. In pressure nozzles the dispersion is obtained by forcing the fluid through a very small orifice at a very high velocity. The pressure nozzles are of two types, single fluid type (e.g. garden hose) and two fluid nozzle type (e.g. perfume atomizer or a paint sprayer). In a single fluid nozzle, the spray is formed by the break-up of the high velocity fluid stream when it comes in contact with the surrounding vapour. In a two fluid atomizing nozzle, the liquid is delivered to the nozzle and dispersed by an impinging stream of gas.

Working

Centrifugal disk atomizers disperse or atomize liquids by spreading them as thin sheets on the disk which are discharged into the surrounding hot gases at high speeds from the periphery of rapidly rotating disks. Centrifugal disk atomization is particularly advantageous for atomizing suspensions and pastes that would clog nozzles or causes excessive erosion.

The contact of the spray and drying medium may be accomplished in a chamber whose shape depends upon the shape of the spray. The centrifugal disk atomizer produces a circular spray with the particles moving in a direction tangential to the circumference of the disk.

Uses

Spray drier is useful if a uniform powdery product is desired. Materials which are heat sensitive are often spray dried as the residence time in the drying chamber is short. The process of spray drying accomplishes both drying and pulverizing in a single step and eliminates the need for a grinding operation that follows other methods of drying. A few products that are dried using spray dryer are: adrenaline, bacitracin, barium sulphate, blood, borax, boric, calcium sulphate, hormones, lactose, methyl cellulose, milk, vitamins and yeast.

Advantages

- Spray drying is a continuous and rapid process. Labour costs are low as many processes like evaporation, crystallization, drying, size reduction and classification takes place at the same time
- Product of uniform and controllable size could be obtained by selecting a suitable atomizer. Uniform free flowing spheres are formed which are very convenient for tableting process
- Fine droplets are formed which provide large surface area for heat and mass transfer. Final product shows excellent solubility
- It is suitable for the drying of sterile products.

Disadvantages

- Equipment is very bulky and expensive
- It is difficult to operate due to huge size
- Low thermal efficiency of dryer as much heat is lost in the discharged gases.

FLUIDIZED BED DRYER (FBD)

Principle

In fluidized bed dryer, fluidization is achieved in a bed of material through vibration or air flow. Then, hot air or combusted gas flow is used to dry powders (direct) or drying takes place through contact with heated surfaces (indirect). An efficient transfer device is created by fluidization which provides intimate contact between each material particle and the gas stream. In fluidised bed dryer, hot air is passed at high pressure though a perforated bottom container containing granules to be dried. The granules are lifted and suspended in the stream of air, this condition is called fluidized state. Every granule is completely dried by the surrounding hot air, ensuring uniformity in drying.

Construction: Two types of fluidized bed dryers are available, vertical fluid bed dryer and horizontal fluid bed dryer.

The construction of a vertical fluidised bed dryer is shown in Fig. 7.6. Stainless steel or plastic is used as material for construction of dryer. A detachable bowl for charging

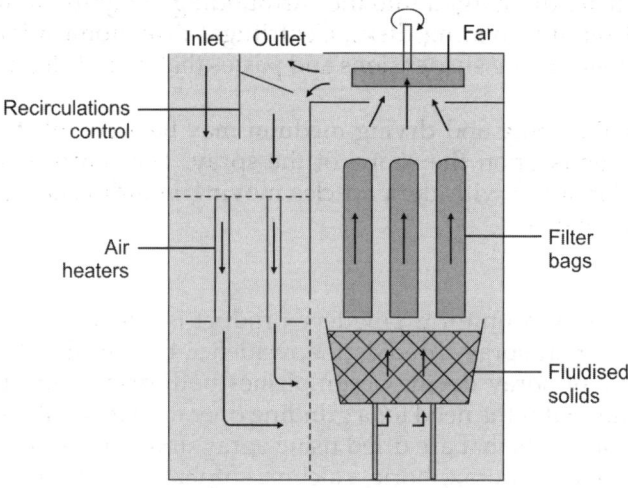

Fig. 7.6: Fluidised bed dryer

and discharging is placed at the bottom of the dryer. The bottom of the bowl is perforated with a wire mesh for placing materials to be dried. A fan is placed in the upper part for circulating hot air. Air is adjusted to desired temperature by fresh air inlet, pre filter and heat exchanger which are connected serially. The temperature of hot air and exit air are monitored. Bag filters are placed above the drying bowl for the recovery of fines which are carried off by the air. Fluidised bed dryer provides good contact between hot air and particles. This technique offers rapid drying and dryers are available in capacities up to 100 kg.

Working: Consider a vessel with perforated base containing particulate matter, the fluid will be able to pass through the bed of solid from below.

If the velocity of the fluid through the bed is increased gradually and the drop in pressure through the bed is measured, a graph is obtained shown in Fig. 7.7.

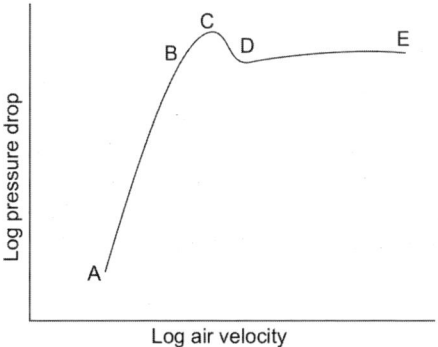

Fig. 7.7: Effect of velocity of air on pressure drop through a fuidized bed

Initially, when the velocity of fluid is low at A aids in smoother and non-turbulent flow of fluids between the particles. Further increase in velocity to point B results in equalization of gravitational force with fraction drag experienced by particle C. The particles try to reduce this resistance by self-rearrangements which leads to suspension of particles in air. The higher porosity D helps to prevent pressure drop of the bed system. A little increment in velocity of fluid there after leads to free movement of separated particles. This stage of bed is regarded as fully fluidized state. Subsequent increase in velocity of fluid up to the point E causes bed expansion devoid of pressure drop, which marks the velocity limit of fluids to suspend the particles.

The total drying time is about 40 minutes. Ambient temperature is achieved by leaving the material in dryer for some time. The bowl is taken out for discharging. The final product is free flowing.

Uses: Fluidized bed dryer is commonly used for drying of granules in the production of tablets. It can also be used for unit operations, such as mixing, granulation and drying. The modified form is used for coating of granules.

Advantages

- Fluidised bed dryer gives drying from individual particles and not from the static bed
- The drying times are shorter than static bed dryers. The dryer has a high output from small floor space
- The temperature of the dryer is uniform and precisely controlled

- The dried product is free flowing
- The drying container is mobile, making handling simple and reducing labour costs
- It facilitates the drying of thermolabile substances, due to short drying time.

Disadvantages

- The fluidized state leads to generation of fines due to turbulence
- Fine materials are collected in filter bags
- Suitable precautions should be taken against the generation of charges of static electricity due to fast movement of particles in hot dry air.

VACUUM DRYER

Principle: In vacuum dryer, drying takes place by the application of vacuum. Due to vacuum, the pressure is lowered so that water boils at a lower temperature resulting in faster evaporation of water.

Construction: Vacuum oven consists of a jacketed vessel strong enough to withstand vacuum within the oven and steam pressure in the jacket. An air-tight seal to the oven is provided by the locked door. The oven is connected through a condenser and receiver to a vacuum pump but the oven can be directly connected to a pump if the liquid which is to be removed is water and pump is of ejector type. The operating pressure of vacuum oven is about 0.03 to 0.06 bar, at this pressure water boils at 25 to 35°C (Fig. 7.8).

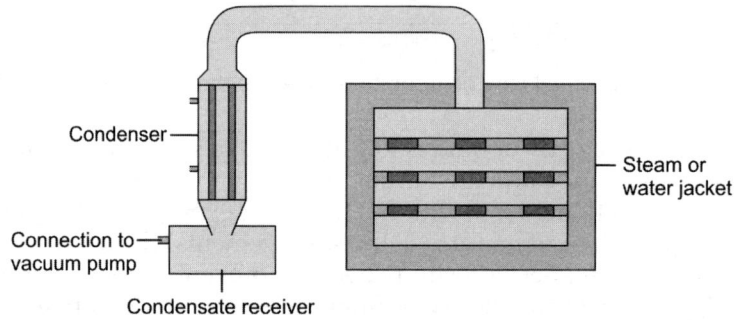

Fig. 7.8: Vacuum dryer

It is possible to recover solvents in a vacuum oven with the help of condenser, which is particularly suitable for expensive or inflammable solvents. This method is advantageous for thermolabile materials, as drying takes place at low temperatures.

Working

For effective conduction heat transfer in vacuum oven, close contact between shelf and tray is required otherwise radiation occurs from the walls and from the shelf above. The capacity of the vacuum dryer could be increased by including an agitator inside the oven so that it can handle large amount of material. The vacuum oven should be checked for excessive temperature gradient as the material thermal conductivity decreases as it get dried which leads to overheating and decomposition.

The material to be dried is spread on trays. The trays are placed on the shelves. Steam or hot air is supplied into the hollow space of jacket and shelves. Heat transfer by conduction takes place. At the end of the drying, vacuum line is disconnected. The material is collected from the trays.

Uses

Application of vacuum drying include preparation of dry extracts where this method of drying produces porous and friable products, when the solvent recovery is advantageous like ethanol derivatives, and drying of thermolabile materials such as penicillin. Dusty and hygroscopic materials and drugs containing toxic and valuable solvents are also dried by this method.

Advantages

- Large surface area for heat transfer is provided in this dryer
- Easier handling of the material, trays and equipment
- It is easy for switching over to the drying of next batches of materials
- Hot water of specified temperatures can be supplied.

Disadvantages

- Heat transfer coefficients are low in vacuum dryer
- It has a limited capacity and used for batch process
- It is more expensive than tray dryer as labour and running costs are also high
- There is a danger of overheating as the material is in contact with steam heated surface for longer period.

FREEZE DRYER

Principle: In freeze drying, the water vapour is sublimed off as frozen material. The structure of material to be dried is better maintained under these conditions. To ensure that sublimation occurs, suitable temperatures and pressures must be maintained in the dryer. To understand this process, the phase diagram for ice-water—water vapour is used to illustrate the interpretation of these diagram for one component system.

In this diagram, each area corresponds to a different phase. The number of degrees of freedom is given by the equation

$$F = 1 - 1 + 2 = 2$$

The temperature and pressure can be varied independently within these areas. If the temperature and pressure is altered, a mass of water under conditions corresponding to point w_1 in Fig. 7.9 may be converted to a mass at higher temperature and pressure at point w_2, that is the number of phases in the system is not altered by the independent variation in temperature and pressure. However, if the conditions are such that the system corresponds to a point that lies on one of the lines AO, BO, or CO, then two phases now exists in equilibrium with each other, since these lines forms the boundaries between different phases. The number of degrees of freedom is reduced, from equation $F = 1 - 2 + 2 = 1$. It means that a single variable exists when equilibrium is established between two phases, and if the pressure is altered, the temperature will assume a definite value or if temperature is altered, the pressure will have a definite value.

Triple Points

The boundary lines meet at O, known as triple point where the three phases may co-exists in equilibrium. The application of phase rule equation to the system at O shows that

$$F = 1 - 3 + 2 = 0$$

It indicates that the system is invariant which means that any change in temperature or pressure will result in alteration of the number of phases.

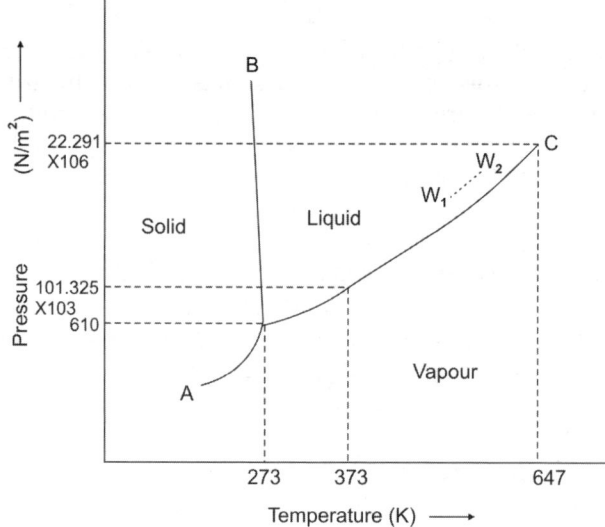

Fig. 7.9: Phase diagram of water at moderate temperature

Sublimation Drying

The line AO, the boundary between vapour and solid phase (known as the sublimation pressure curve for ice) represents the coexistence of vapour and solid phases in equilibrium. A mass of ice may be converted directly into water vapour by heating, provided the pressure is below the triple point pressure. Removal of water by means of sublimation is known as sublimation or freeze drying and is relevant in drying compounds that are sensitive to higher temperatures.

Construction: The construction of a freeze dryer is shown in Fig. 7.10. It consists of:
- Drying chamber in which trays are loaded
- Heat coils to supply heat in the form of radiation source
- Vapour condensing or adsorption system
- Vacuum pump or steam ejector or both.

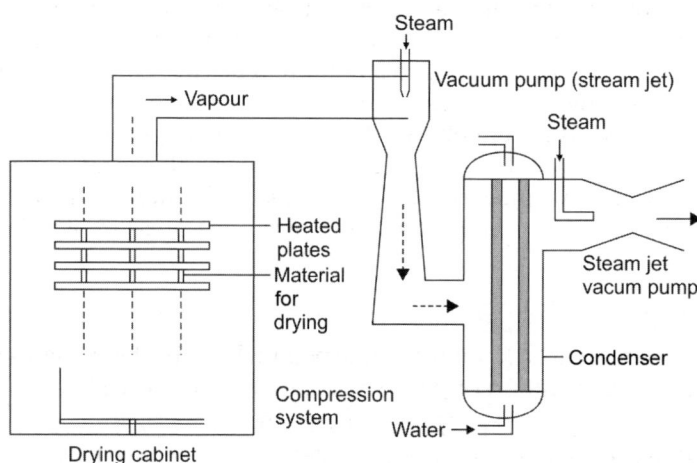

Fig. 7.10: Freeze dryer

The chamber for vacuum drying consists of shelves for keeping the material. The distance between subliming surface and condenser must be less than the mean path of molecules which increases the rate of drying. The condenser consists of a relatively large surface cooled by solid carbon dioxide slurred with acetone or ethanol. The temperature of the condenser must be much lower than the evaporated surface of frozen substance.

Working

Freeze drying or sublimation drying consists of reducing the temperature and pressure to values below the triple point. The temperature must be below the triple point, and usually – 10 to – 30°C is employed. Similarly, the pressure will be below the triple point and pressures between 10 and 30 N/m^2 are generally used.

- Stages of freeze drying:
  - Pre-freezing
  - Primary drying
  - Secondary drying
  - Packaging.

Pre-freezing

The solution can be pre-frozen before the beginning of drying process. In shell freezing, the bottle is partly filled up with the product and is placed horizontally and slowly rotated in a refrigerated bath. This would increase area for heat transfer during drying. In vertical spin freezing method, the bottles are first chilled and then spun in vertical position in a stream of very cold air. Freezing occurs very rapidly, liquid become super-cooled and small crystals of ice are formed.

Primary Drying

In this step, the latent heat of sublimation must be provided to the material and the vapour removed. Heat transfer is critical at this stage. Insufficient heat prolongs the process and excess heat may cause melting. During the process, vapours are formed which must be removed continuously to avoid a pressure rise that would stop sublimation. For small scale operations, vapours are absorbed by a desiccant such as phosphorous pentaoxide or are cooled on a small condenser with solid carbon dioxide. For large scale, mechanically refrigerated condensers are used. On the large scale, vapour is commonly removed by ejector pump which could handle large amount of vapours and is not affected by moisture. The rate of drying in freeze drying is very low, of the order of 1 mm per hour. The mechanism of freeze drying represents the falling rate period of the usual drying process.

Secondary Drying

At the end of primary drying process, about 0.5% of moisture is left in the solid and this amount has to be removed during secondary drying process. Secondary drying is a vacuum drying process whereas the product contains negligible amount of moisture, risk of hydrolysis is minimal.

Packaging

The freeze dried products are packaged taking care to ensure protection from moisture.

Advances in freeze drying

One innovation has been radiant heating with infrared bulbs or a dielectric heater inside the freeze dryer. The costs and time required to sublime the material is reduced by using dielectric heaters wherein dielectric heat is produced internally in the frozen portion of the specimen. Other advancement is use of microwave to induce microwave vibrations (microwaves freeze drying).

Advantages

- The hydrolytic degradation is minimized due to low temperature drying. Under high vacuum there is no contact with air and hence oxidative degradation is also minimized
- Volume of dried product is same as the original solution, thus there is no case hardening and the product is light and porous. The porous product gives ready solubility
- There is no concentration of the solution before drying. Hence, salts do not concentrate and denature proteins
- Migration of salts and other solutes does not take place
- Loss of volatile material is less
- Low moisture level can be maintained without decomposition
- Material can be dried in its final container like single dose and multiple dose vials
- Sterility can be maintained
- The final product can be stored at ambient temperature in inert atmosphere.

Disadvantages

- The freeze drying process being very slow and expensive is limited to valuable products which cannot be dried by other means
- The product obtained is very hygroscopic which needs special packaging
- Equipment and running costs are high.

Uses

This process is applied to biological products; antibiotics (other than penicillin), blood products, vaccines (such as BCG, yellow fever, smallpox), enzyme preparations (hyaluronidase) and microbiological cultures, bacterial and viral cultures, human tissue (arteries and corneal tissue), antibiotics and plant extracts, steroids, vitamins and enzymes.

VERY SHORT QUESTIONS

1. **Differentiate between drying and evaporation.**

2. **Name suitable dryers.**
   a. Granular free flowing solids
   b. Wet bricks before sending to kilns
   c. Sticky paste
   d. Food products like horlicks

3. **Explain critical moisture content and equilibrium moisture content.**

4. **Define bound moisture and free moisture content.**

5. Give the factors affecting constant drying rate.

6. List the critical conditions for drying of various substances.

7. Define drying. Give its importance's in the formulation of dosage forms.

8. Describe mechanism of drying.

9. How will you obtained the rate of drying curve for a given drying operation? Give its applications.

SHORT QUESTIONS

1. Give classification of dryers with suitable examples.

2. Name a suitable dryer for drying the following substances and substantiate your answer with at least two reasons.
   a. Liver extracts
   b. Granular solids
   c. Pasty materials
   d. Granules of heat sensitive drugs
   e. Vitamin B complex granules
   f. Colloidal solution

3. Explain the drying rate curve for a non-porous granular solid and crude fibrous drug.

4. Give the principle and enlist the pharmaceutical application with the help of a labelled diagram of fluidized bed dryer.

5. Explain the principle of spray drying with suitable labelled diagram.

6. Describe the drying rate curve. Explain its applications.

7. Explain the principles and working of freeze dryer.

8. Differentiate spray drying with drying in a vacuum shell dryer.

9. Compare the operations of spray dryer and tray dryer.

10. Describe the concept of vacuum dryer. What are its advantages? Compare the spray drying with other methods of drying?

LONG QUESTIONS

1. Describe the construction operational details of freeze dryer. Describe its application in pharmacy.

2. Explain the concept of spray drying. Describe the specific advantages of spray dried product over drum dried material. Also list the pharmaceutical applications.

3. Classify dryers. Describe in detail the constant rate and falling rate periods. Add a note on critical moisture content.

4. For drying of milk which dryer is used drum dryers or spray dryers. Which dryer will you prefer and why? Discuss freeze dryer in detail.

5. Discuss the construction, working, advantages and disadvantages of spray dryer.

6. Explain the theory behind drying and rate of drying with suitable graphs.

MULTIPLE CHOICE QUESTIONS

1. This initial drying period is followed by a much slower rate of drying as the moisture content of the product ....
   a. Decrease
   b. Increase
   c. Constant
   d. None of above

2. State why direct heating by hot air cannot be done in some cases?
   a. The material can degrade
   b. High temperature not required
   c. Low temperature not required
   d. Conduction gives best results

3. When are drum dryers used?
   a. When the material is too thick for spray dryer and too thin for rotary dryer
   b. When the material is too thick for rotary dryer and too thin for spray dryer
   c. When the material is not biodegradable
   d. When large crystal size is to be obtained

4. How is heating achieved in drum dryers?
   a. By heating the drums
   b. By conduction
   c. By passing steam through hollow screws
   d. By passing steam through the conveyer belt

5. Which materials are not used in drying in a freeze dryer?
   a. Seafood
   b. Fruits
   c. Pharmaceuticals
   d. Dyes

6. How the liquid does gets separated in freeze dryer?
   a. Boiling
   b. Distillation
   c. Freezing and crystallization
   d. Evaporation

7. Heat sensitive or easily oxidizable materials are dried by:
   a. Flash dryer
   b. Drum dryer
   c. Fluidized bed dryer
   d. Rotary dryer

8. With what is the feed introduced in the spary dryer?
   a. Spray
   b. Atomizer
   c. Nucleator
   d. Heat exchanger

9. What is the use of a high pressure nozzle or a whirling disk in a spray dryer?
   a. Increasing contact time
   b. Decreasing contact time
   c. Agitation
   d. Atomization

10. Which dryer used radiation for drying?
    a. Spray dryer
    b. Drum dryer
    c. Flash dryer
    d. Microwave dryer

11. **What is the drum dryer called if it is open to the atmosphere?**
    a. Open dryer   b. Box dryer
    c. Trough dryer   d. Trench dryer

12. **Direct dryers are known as:**
    a. Batch dryers   b. Continuous dryers
    c. Semi-batch dryers   d. None of the mentioned

13. **Cabinet/Tray driers are direct driers.**
    a. True   b.   False

14. **For estimating the drier size it is necessary to know ....**
    a. Time of drying   b. Heat of drying
    c. Speed of drying   d. All of the mentioned

15. **For a batch drying, the wet surface should be more compare to dry surface.**
    a. True   b.   False

16. **Find the missing position.**

    a. Time   b. Speed
    c. Water vapour   d. None of the above

17. **After the unsaturated drying completed .... starts to evaporate.**
    a. Bound   b. Unbound
    c. Equilibrium   d. None of the above

18. **The other part than the constant rate period in the Batch-Drying curve is falling rate period.**
    a. True
    b. False

19. **The value of .... remains constant while drying if speed and direction of gas flow never changes.**
    a. Mass transfer coefficient
    b. Humidity
    c. Moisture
    d. None of above

20. **Constant drying conditions includes:**
    a. Temperature constant
    b. Humidity constant
    c. Velocity constant
    d. All of the mentioned

21. **If the dry spot appears in the substance in the batch drying curve at** ....
    a. Critical moisture content
    b. Equilibrium moisture content
    c. Bound moisture
    d. Unbound moisture

22. **After critical moisture content** .... **starts.**
    a. Saturated drying region
    b. Unsaturated drying region
    c. Constant drying region
    d. None of the mentioned

8

Mixing

Saima Amin, Atefeh A Mogaddam and Yasmin Sultana

Mixing is the state that results in randomization of different particles inside a system into a uniform product in which there is a possibility of finding the particles of the added ingredients same at all points in the mixture to ensure the uniform distribution of the active ingredient. Although it is the method of thoroughly combining different materials to produce a homogeneous product but it is also to allow heat and/or mass transfer to occur between one or more streams, components or phases. Mixing is one of the most frequently and widely used unit operation in pharmaceutical engineering. It is usually used when a product contains more than one ingredient.

Mixing is a critical process as the quality of the mixture determines the quality of the final product. Inappropriate mixing ends in a non-homogeneous product that lacks uniformity with respect to desired characteristics like particle size, chemical composition, colour and flavour. In the initial stages of mixing process the rate of mixing is very fast as the mixing elements change their circulation path rapidly while they discover themselves in different situations, whereas the rate of mixing at the final step of the process becomes nearly zero as particles do not find different situations.

APPLICATIONS

- It is used to blend different components in order to ensure even distribution of drug in a dosage form and to attain even appearance
- It helps in preparations of formulations, such as of solid particles example tablets, capsules, inhalers, sachets
- It is widely applicable in miscible liquids dosage form preparation, such as linctuses, solutions
- Apart from simple combination of raw components, mixing accomplishes preparations of several formulations of immiscible liquids, such as suspensions, fine emulsions, pastes and creams
- It enables heat transfer and dissolving ingredients
- It helps in reducing particle size, augmenting chemical reactions and also in controlling rheology
- The mixing operation has a definite influence on whether a drug will have an acceptable form and consistency to deliver the accurate dose to the targeted site
- It helps in attaining drug stablity for the appropriate duration of time

- Uniform mixing of dosage forms helps the manufacturer to enable product as a single phase system
- Its control is also important in other unit operations, such as drying, granulation and coating.

OBJECTIVES OF MIXING

The most important objectives of the mixing can be classified as:

- The first and foremost objective of mixing is to produce a simple physical mixture of two or more miscible liquids or uniformly divided solids to bring them into a uniform product
- Achievement of complete and uniform distribution of the component materials throughout the whole mixture is yet another objective of mixing
- To produce a physical change in the ingredient that is used in building-up of pharmaceuticals
- Producing a dispersion of two immiscible liquids into an emulsion or a suspension
- To assure and control a chemical reaction by increasing the contact surface between the components thus promoting chemical and physical reactions to produce a uniform product.

FACTORS AFFECTING MIXING

There are several factors that affect the mixing process. Some of the crucial factors are discussed below:

- **Trough size and shape:** The various mixing vessels are designed in such a way that material to fill capacity ratio of the vessel is optimal to allow maximum blending or shearing. Also the position of the shaft is important which ensures proper movement of the blades attached. For example, in Ribbon blenders, the trough is filled with 40–70% of the total volume of the trough for efficient mixing; therefore size of the vessel is important. The shape of the vessels also affects the efficiency of most of the mixers, e.g. round vessels are better than square ones in propeller mixers.

- **Nature of the product:** Materials with oppositely charged particles have a tendency to adhere to the carrier, the vessel. Also, these charged particles do cling to metal parts, such as blade, propellers, etc. thus causing further segregation of material. Humid material is less conductive thus leads to inefficient mixing. Flaky particles as in hulls are difficult to handle because they interlock and form obstructions to flow. If particles of the material are light, these are nuisance, a safety hazard and indicate potential loss of micro-ingredients into the air. Therefore, for such particles, dust collection system is required. The manufacturers are required to perform analyses regularly on dust to determine which specific active ingredients are present and at what levels. These dust particles are responsible for carry-over and contamination. If a material is hygroscopic, a significant uptake of moisture can result in change in a number of physical properties, such as caking or clumping, reduction in particle numbers, increased particle size and density. This hampers uniformity in the mix. Free-flowing materials offer effective blending with unrealistic processing costs. Factors, such as particle size and shape, bulk density, hygroscopicity and electrostatic charge affect flowability.

- **Particle size:** Uniform sized particles in a mixture ends up in a uniform blend. Non-uniform sized particles result in separation of particles as the small particles move downward between the bigger particles through the spaces. Also the influence of gravitational force on the size can be described as flow properties increase as the particle size increases.

- **Particle shape:** Ingredients with spherical shapes are more suitable for uniform mixing. The particles with irregular shapes can lead to interlocking and there are less chances of ingredient separation once they are mixed together.

- **Density:** The difference in densities of the mixed particles leads to segregation. The heavy particles settle down and sediment while the lighter ones occupy the upper space thus making two different phases. Mixed particles must be equal in density to achieve good mixing. The degree of mixing increases slowly until equilibrium is achieved. Usually, the heavier particles form the lower layer in a mixture. And if the heavier component is at the top, the degree of mixing rises to a maximum level and then follows equilibrium which is due to dropping of the heavier ingredients through the lighter one.

- **Electrostatic charges:** Due to stirring and mixing of the components, constant friction among the mixed particles and between particles and the wall of the container, leads to formation of electronic charges. Generally, the most severe electrostatic charge is carried by fine powder particles. The high surface area can lead to high charging levels, with coarser particles carrying less charge.

  Similar charges keep away particles from each other, leading to separation of particles. This can be overcome by adding surfactants (surface active agent) or wetting agents to reduce the surface tension of the particles to neutralize similar developed charges on the particles. In solid mixing, adding some amount of water and evaporating it after mixing leads to reduction in electrostatic charges.

- **Proportions of materials to be mixed:** This property plays a crucial role in solid mixing. Mixing equal amount of powders is easier than mixing small quantities of powder (potent powder) with different amount of other ingredients. When more than two ingredients are going to be mixed they are required to be added in ascending order of their weights to attain uniform mixing of the components.

CLASSIFICATION OF MIXTURES

A mixture is a product of mechanical blending or mixing of chemical substances, such as compounds which are the combination of two or more different substances without chemical changes or chemical bonding, so that each substance maintains its own chemical properties which can usually be separated by non-chemical means. They can be classified into three types depending upon the way they combine with other particles; suspension, colloidal and solution.

  i. **Suspensions** are the mixtures which have larger particles above 1 micron meter with heterogeneous look.

  ii. **Colloidal** mixtures have much smaller particles ranging from 1 nm- 1 micron meter and they look visually homogeneous but appear in different sizes under microscope.

  iii. **Solutions** are the mixture in which particles are completely dissolved into the solvent and the final product looks homogeneous.

Mixtures can also be classified as homogeneous or heterogeneous mixtures:

  i. **Homogeneous** mixture is a mixture in which every part of the solution has same properties as others and the composition of final product is uniform.

  ii. **Heterogeneous** mixture is a mixture in which the constituents can be seen due to the presence of two or more phases.

Mixtures may also be Classified as

Positive Mixtures

These types of mixtures are formed by spontaneous mixing of two or more gases or miscible liquids by means of diffusion process. It results in an irreversible mixing but a perfect mix. No input of energy in this process is required and the time allowed for solution formation is highly sufficient, e.g. alcohol in water or sugar in water.

Negative Mixtures

These mixtures are formed when insoluble solids are mixed with a vehicle (e.g. suspension) or when immiscible liquids are mixed (e.g. emulsion) and require energy for their formulation. They are generally very difficult to form and require a high degree of mixing efficiency to remain stable, e.g. mixing of two immiscible liquids to form an emulsion or insoluble solids with a vehicle to form a suspension.

Neutral Mixtures

They are static in their behaviour and the components of such types of product do not have a tendency to mix or segregate spontaneously but once they are mixed, they do not separate out easily unless a force is applied on the system, e.g. of neutral mixtures include ointments, mixed powders and paste.

TYPES OF MIXING

Solid-solid Mixing (Powder Mixing)

The mixing of solids is one of the most common pharmaceutical operations and is a critically important procedure in processes where the active ingredient in a formulation may be toxic and needs to be present at a low concentration that too uniformly blended with adjuvants. When the dose of the active substance is high, mixing is not a problem. A product with very low active ingredient will become an ineffective compound and while a product with too high active ingredients may become lethal.

Segregation is a phenomenon related to particle's tendency owing to size, shape, density, etc.

It needs to be prevented or overcome to provide final good solid mixing.

Mechanism of Solid Mixing

Segregation phenomenon of particles can occur due to a number of reasons which mixing can avoid. There are three main principal mechanisms in solid-solid mixing to describe mixing performance. These are convective mixing, shear mixing and diffusive mixing.

Convective mixing

Convective mixing is achieved by the transport of the powder components using blades, paddles or screw element for a large mass of material transport from one part to another. It is also referred as macromixing.

Shear Mixing

As the forces of attraction between the particles are broken down, each particle moves on its own between areas of different ingredient and parallel to their surfaces. This leads to shear mixing.

Diffusive Mixing

Diffusive mixing refers to random movement of particles within the powder bed by diffusion process, so particles change their places relative to one another. Sometimes it is referred as micromixing.

Mechanism of Liquid-liquid Mixing

The mechanism for fluid mixing, which involves two liquids include:

a. **Bulk transport:** In this transport, there is movement of large portion of material from one location to another location. Rotating blades and paddles are used in this system.

b. **Turbulent mixing:** It is a highly effective procedure and mixing is due to turbulent flow that results in random oscillation of the fluid speed at any given point within the system and the speed of the fluid at a given point changes in three directions (X, Y and Z).

Laminar Mixing

The principle is mixing of two different liquids through laminar flow, i.e. applied shear gives the interface between them. It is suitable for liquids which require adequate mixing.

Molecular Diffusion

In this system the mixing happens at molecular level in which molecules diffuse due to thermal motion.

MECHANISM OF SEMISOLIDS MIXING

Semisolids dosage forms include ointments, pastes, creams, jellies, etc. The mixing action includes combination of low speed shear, rubbing, wiping, folding, stretching and compressing. The mechanism involving mixing of semisolids depends on the character of the materials that shows considerable variation. Semisolids form neutral mixture because they have no tendency to segregate. The mixers for mixing the semi-solids must have rotating elements with narrow clearances between themselves and the mixing vessel wall and they must produce a high degree of shear mixing, so that diffusion and convection cannot occur.

In semisolid mixing moving parts of the vessels exert great amount of mechanical energy to the material which results in heat as well as high power consumption. Therefore, it is required that the equipment must have a coarse surface to withstand these forces. Some semisolid materials show dilatant property, i.e. their viscosity increases with rise in shear rates, thus mixing of such materials should be completed at low speeds. The speed of unit operation must be changed while handling thixotropic, plastic and pseudoplastic materials.

DIFFERENCE BETWEEN SOLID AND LIQUID MIXING

In general, powders are neutral mixtures. In liquids, the mixed condition is not difficult to achieve with two or more mobile liquids.

Flow currents exists in liquid mixing which transport unmixed liquid close to the impeller for effective mixing, but no such flow currents exists in solid mixing. Large sample size is required to evaluate the extent of solid mixing but, a small sample is enough to examine liquid mixing. Power requirement is high for solid mixing but less for liquid mixing.

EQUIPMENT USED FOR MIXING

Different range of equipment is used in pharmaceutical production of different dosage forms. In some of these equipment the container rotates while in others the container is stationary but a device rotates inside that. Other containers are available which have both rotating containers and internal device (Fig. 8.1). Manual operated mixers include:

Pestle and Mortar

Pestle and mortar is a traditional and simplest equipment for crushing and mixing. In this process, the material is grinded and mixed by applying abrasion and pressure.

Spatula

A spatula is a broad, flat, flexible metallic blade used to mix dry powder materials. It is derived from Latin word for a flat piece of wood. It is used to blend powders in small quantities.

Sieves

Sieve is a woven mesh assembly used to mix the material through sifting. It is an oldest and convenient method of mixing the powders.

Power Operated Equipment

Agitator Mixers

Agitator mixers are similar to paddle mixers used for liquids, however their efficiency is low. In this type the main container is non-rotating but the internal blade is moving and creating planetary motion which is highly effective. They are commonly available

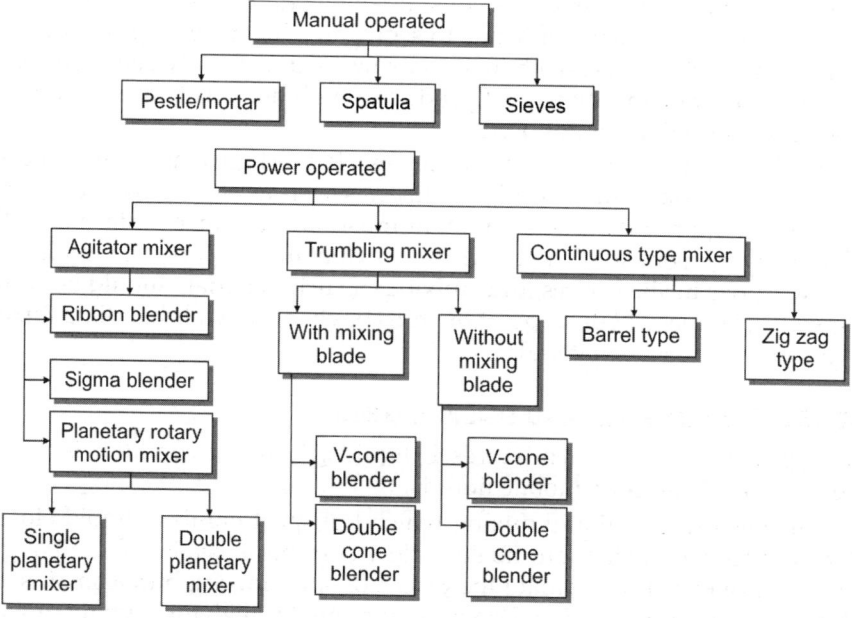

Fig. 8.1: Different categories of equipment used in mixing

in the form of rack having an internal arm that rotates and transfers shearing forces to the particles. Due to the two-dimensional shear forces in these mixers, aggregates may stay unbroken followed by the slow movement of the blade which may encourage segregation due to density or size differences of the particles. This type of mixer is most appropriate for components with uniform size and density and for mixing free-flowing materials. These are of three types: ribbon, sigma and planetary mixers.

Tumbling Mixers

In this mixer, rotation of the vessel causes movement to the materials. Here mixing is done by tumbling motion, which is accentuated by shape of the container. Simple forms rotate on their horizontal axis using a cylindrical vessel but have low shear forces and end-to-end movement is minor. Vessel is mounted on special roller so that it can be rotated about any axis. This may be avoided by introducing a form of baffles, or the shape of the container that may be change to avoid symmetry. This shape gives effective 3D shearing and movement occurs as the material flows. Due to considerable velocity and acceleration gradients the particles hit against the container's wall and are bounced. The tumbling mixers preferable as repeated reversal of the direction of flow makes differences in density of particle size to occur. Rate of rotation depends upon nature of the material to be mixed, size of particles and shape of the tumbler.

Continuous Type

In continuous mixers, material flows steadily into the mixer, and then is retained in the mixing vessel for a specified mixing time. The discharge occurs at the same flow rate. These mixers offer higher processing capacities without variation in mixing. Continuous mixers are used to mix ingredients continuously in a mixer in a single pass. In a continuous mixing process, weighing, loading, mixing and discharge steps occur continuously and simultaneously.

SOME SPECIFIC MIXERS ARE DISCUSSED BELOW

DOUBLE CONE BLENDER

It is an efficient and versatile machine for mixing of dry powders and granules homogeneously. They are most often used for dry blending of free flowing solids. The solids being blended in these units can vary in bulk density and in percentage of the total mixture. Materials being blended are constantly being intermixed as the double cone rotates.

Principle: The principle behind mixing in a double cone blender is the diffusion process, where small scale random motion of solid particles occurs. The blend in the equipment offers high mobility of particles leading to diffusive blending where the particles are distributed over a freshly developed interface. In it, bulk transport and shear which occur due to tumbling are responsible for mixing of solid.

Construction: It consists of hollow cylindrical shell made-up of stainless steel, i.e. mounted on a shaft that helps to tumble the contents placed in blender, i.e. driven by shaft drive. It is usually charged and discharged through the same port. It is an efficient design for mixing contents of different densities. The rate of rotation should be optimum depending upon the size and shape of the tumbler and also on nature of material required to be mixed. Normal cycle time is typically in the range of 10 minutes, at 30 to 100 rpm. However, it can be less depending on the difficulty of blending (Fig. 8.2).

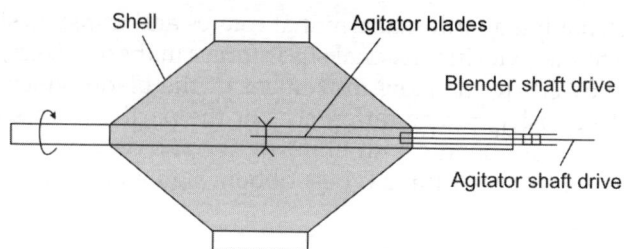

Shell   Agitator blades

Blender shaft drive

Agitator shaft drive

Fig. 8.2: Double cone blender rotating shell with rotating baffles

Working: The material to be mixed is charged into the vessel through the ends of either cylinder or through the open port. The blending efficiency is affected by the fill volume. The effective volume for optimum homogeneity is between 35 and 70% of gross volume. If the volume of the material is increased to 70%, the time for blending is doubled. The blender speed plays a vital role in mixing efficiency. Low speed offers low shear forces but high speed provides high shear forces leading to separation of fines which then settle at the top of the blender when it is stopped. Also if shear rotation is too high then powder bed experiences centrifugal force and again the efficiency of mixing decreases. Usually, these blends are constructed to operate at 50–80% of the critical speed. The blended material is discharged through the open port fitted with a discharge valve.

Applications

- It is used for tablets and capsules formulations
- It is used in preparation of dry granules to increase the batch size at bulk lubrication stage of tablet granules
- It is used for dry powder mixing
- It is used in pharmaceuticals, foods, chemicals, fertilizers, plastics, pigments, cosmetics and industries.

Advantages

- It is used for fragile materials as there is no blade present which can cause attrition
- Charging the material into the apparatus and its removal is easy
- There are least chances of contamination
- Easy to clean
- The conical shape at both ends enables uniform mixing and easy discharge
- Suitable size for material discharge and hole with openable cover provided at other end of the cone for material charging
- Capacities available are 20 to 3000 L.

Disadvantages

- The mixer is not suitable for variable size and density of powder as segregation can occur
- Large space is required for installation.

TWIN SHELL BLENDER

It is also called V-blender. It is used for mixing process where precise blend formulation is required. They are also used where the ingredients are less than 5% of the total bulk.

The operation is completed within 5 to 15 minutes depending upon the properties of the materials to be used. Here the container is mobile.

Principle: The principle behind mixing in a twin shell blender is the diffusion process, where small scale random motion of solid particles occurs. The blend in the equipment offers high mobility of particles leading to diffusive blending where the particles are distributed over a freshly developed interface. In twin shell blender, bulk transport and shear which occur due to tumbling are responsible for mixing of solid.

Construction: Twin shell blender consists of two hollow cylindrical shells joined at an angle of 75 to 90°. The container is then mounted on a rod to allow the hollow cylinders to tumble. Here the material placed in the blender is constantly split and recombined and thorough mixing occurs. Due to repetitive converging and diverging motion, along with frictional forces between the material and vessel it lead to homogeneous mixing (Fig. 8.3).

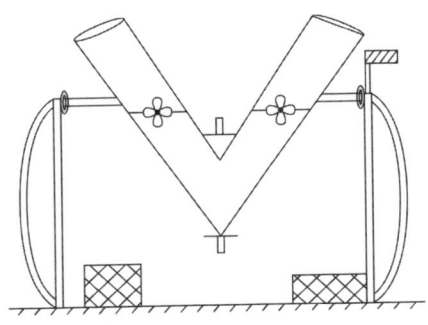

Fig. 8.3: Twin shell blender

Working: The material to be mixed is charged into the vessel through the ends of either cylinder or through the open port. The blending efficiency is affected by the fill volume. Usually 50–60% of the total blender volume is occupied by the material. If the volume of the material is increased to 70%, the time for blending is doubled. The blender speed plays a vital role in mixing efficiency. Low speed offers low shear forces but high speed provides high shear forces leading to separation of fines which then settle at the top of the blender when it is stopped. Also if shear rotation is too high then powder bed experiences centrifugal force and again the efficiency of mixing decreases. Every V-blender has a critical speed which means when a blend reaches the critical speed, its efficiency decreases. Usually, these blends are constructed to operate at 50–80% of the critical speed. The blended material is discharged through the open port fitted with a discharge valve.

Applications
- It is good for dry as well as wet mixing
- The equipment is suitable for handling fine and coarse powders.

Advantages
- It is used for fragile materials as there is no blade present which can cause attrition
- Charging the material into the apparatus and its removal is easy
- There are least chances of contamination
- Easy to clean.

Disadvantages

- The mixer is not suitable for variable size and density of powder as segregation can occur.
- Large space is required for installation.

RIBBON BLENDERS

Ribbon blenders are the mixing devices used for mixing of powder with cohesiveness.

Principle: Ribbon blender works on the principle of radial movement caused by the rotation of the ribbons. Axial movement is also induced due to difference in the peripheral speeds of the outer and the inner ribbons. The amalgamation of radial and axial movement results in homogeneous mixing within 15 to 20 minutes.

Construction: Ribbon blender consists of a U-shaped trough to hold the material. There is a double helical ribbon agitator that rotates within the trough. The shaft is positioned in the centre of the trough to which helical ribbons are attached. Since, the ribbon agitator has inner and outer helical ribbons, it is also called double helical ribbon agitator. There is a narrow gap of 3–6 mm between the agitator and the inner wall of the trough (Fig. 8.4).

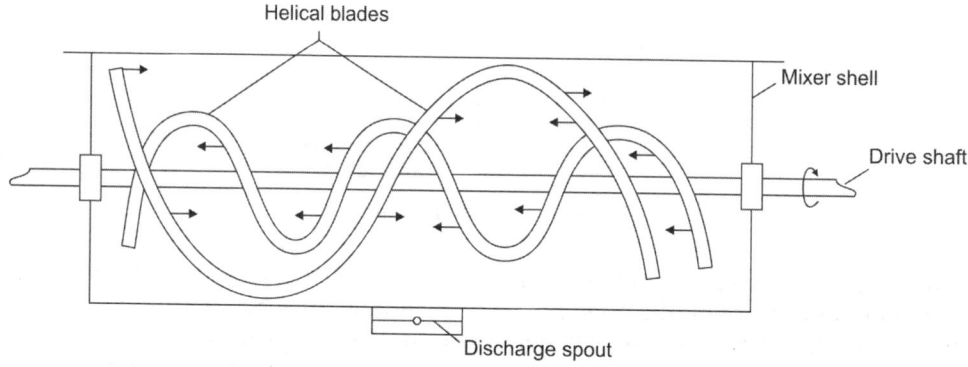

Fig. 8.4: Ribbon blender

Working: Ribbon blender is operated through power system at 10–15 horse power. End plates are tightly screwed or welded to the U-shaped container and have exit for the shaft thus, the material inside the container does not travel. There is a feed hopper or the top cover to allow changing of material. An external jacket is also provided to the equipment for blending of materials which require heat/temperature maintenance. Usually, the blender is filled with 40–70% of the total volume of the trough. A spray pipe is mounted on the top cover for adding liquids. Also high speed chopper is assembled inside the trough to rupture the agglomerates. The discharge valve located at the bottom of the trough allows the discharge of the blended material. These valves can be operated manually or actuated pneumatically. The discharge of the material is attained by rotation of the agitator therefore 100% discharge is not possible like in other blenders.

Applications

- Ribbon blenders are widely used in pharmaceuticals for coating, blending and drying of powder/particles
- They are used for blending of cosmetic powders

- Before filling of powder into capsules, the blend of different ingredients is mixed through ribbon blenders.

Advantages
- Ribbon blender offers mixing of dry solids
- They are used to coat solid particles with small amount of liquids
- Ribbon blenders are used for lubrication of dry granules and bulk mixing of drugs
- Friable material is also blended, provided a paddle design is used instead of ribbons
- They offer fast mixing of materials with different physical properties
- Since, the equipment has lower height, so its installation is easy
- The two ribbons (positive and negative) are set at the same level therefore, mixing with high efficiency and low power consumption is attained
- Since, the apparatus is operated at a critical speed, therefore effect of fragmentation is reduced.

Disadvantages
- Regions of high shear or pinch points are developed which damage the fragile material
- Due to this heat is also generated leading to degradation of product
- The unmixed spots at the bottom of trough pose problem in discharge.

SIGMA MIXERS
Sigma mixers are the commonly used mixers for handling high viscous materials, such as adhesives, rubber, etc. They are also called double arm kneader mixer.

Principle: Sigma mixers are operated on a principle to promote lateral and transverse motion.

Construction: Sigma mixers consist of a trough which is a W-shaped container. There are two mixing blades which operate at a same or variable speed to ensure proper kneading of material. The blades which are used in the mixer are sigma blade, shredder blade, spiral blade or the masticator blade. The material is loaded in trough to 40–65% of the total volume capacity of the mixer. Also the blades are operated at a close clearance of 2–3 mm (Fig. 8.5).

Working: In sigma blenders, the blades are rotated either tangentially to each other where the front blade rotates faster than the rear blade with a speed ratio of 3:2, or are overlapped within the trough. Here the relative position of the blades is unchanged

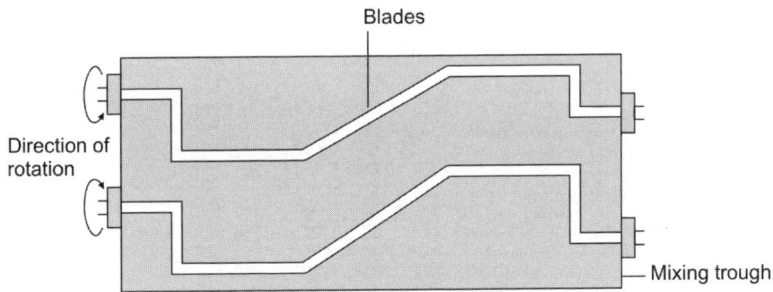

Fig. 8.5: Sigma blade mixer

thus, they are operated at the same speed. Also the blades are operated at a close clearance of 2–3 mm which means the blades pass the container wall and each other very closely therefore, allowing homogeneous mixing. The rotation of the blade is carried out through drive system consists of gearbox, couplings and gears. For the control of temperature, water jacket is provided to the mixer otherwise it can be operated at ambient temperature. Discharge of the material occurs by tilting the trough or through discharge valve at the bottom of the vessel. In some models, extruder/ screw discharge valve is located at the bottom where the two trough compartment meets. It has the advantage of delivering the material of desired shape and size.

Applications
- Sigma blender is used for mixing of pasty material
- High viscosity material is mixed and kneaded.

Advantages
- High viscosity materials are handled efficiently
- Mixing homogeneity of 99% is attained
- Mixing is achieved within 10–30 minutes
- Consistent particle size distribution is produced without the provision of choppers.

Disadvantages
- High power consumption
- High fill volume is not possible.

PLANETARY MIXER

Though newer technologies in mixing have come up with single pot processing but still pharmaceutical industry is relying on planetary mixers for blending viscous ingredients. Planetary mixers are widely used for lab scale to large scale production. They offer quick, intensive, homogeneous and dead spot free mixing (Fig. 8.6).

Principle: Planetary mixer offers planetary motion. While being revolved around central axis the agitators rotate on their own axis, thus generating planetary motion. The planetary mixers are based on the principle of laminar mixing where the two dissimilar liquids result in increase in interfacial area as a result of stretching and thinning of the layer of material.

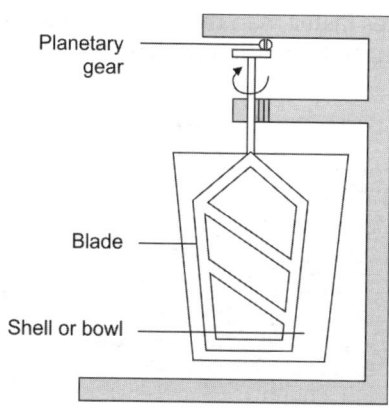

Planetary gear

Blade

Shell or bowl

Fig. 8.6: Planetary mixer

Construction: Planetary mixer consists of a mixing bowl which holds the material. It is made of stainless steel as per cGMP requirements. The bowl of the single planetary mixer consists of an upper cylindrical section and a lower hemispherical section. The mixer bowl is secured to a semi-circular frame (also called fork) at the time of mixing. The bigger models have the container fixed to the bottom or are provided with wheels mounted at the bottom for easy mobility. The design of a beater is selected to match the lower curved surface of the bowl. The beater is usually two in numbers that offers two types of movements. It revolves on its own vertical axis at high speed and at the same time, this vertical axis rotates around the centre of the bowl at lower speed. The two mixing blades, each of which is mounted on a unique axis which in turn is attached to a joint axis allowing the blades to exhibit same movement apart from their individual movement. And to sweep the entire inner lining of the vessel, the blades revolve in opposite direction. A high speed emulsifier called homogenizer is also provided at the centre axis. The homogenizer offers blending of material due to ex-centric movement of the product. The bigger models are also provided with motorized system for mixing drives to offer up and down movement of the blades. The removable bowl design allows mixing of large number of batches with minimum loss of production. To improve the efficiency of the operation, usually one bowl is attached to the mixer (in operation) while the other bowl is loaded with material to be mixed for the next batch. Planetary mixers operate on the planetary motion of the beater used for blending the material in the bowl. The blending occurs without dead spaces. Sometimes, scrapers with Teflon edges may also be provided to wipe any material that may stick to the inner surface of the container. The mixing bowl of a planetary mixer can also be electric/steam jacketed for mixing viscous materials. The top of the vessel is covered with a lid which has a charging hole to feed the material into the bowl. A discharge valve is present at the bottom for material discharge. A platen style hydraulic discharge system offers speedy discharge of material and cleaning of the vessel.

Once the process is complete, the bowl is lowered and then detached from the mixer assembly. The lifting and lowering of the bowl is done manually in small size mixers however in larger mixers, either the bowl is lowered with the help of a motor or the beater is raised above the bowl, using a motorized or hydraulically operated mechanical arrangement. The bowl is then moved away from the machine using trolley with wheels, called dolly.

Double planetary mixer is also constructed for handling high viscosity material. These mixers have a rectangular stirrer or high viscosity blade which generates vertical mixing due to its angled helical contour. Thus problem of climbing which occurs with high filled materials is solved. The blades run at a high speed thus are less sensitive to shifts in viscosity when liquid is added.

Applications

- Planetary mixers are used for wet/dry material
- They are used to manufacture pastes of starch with steam jacketed vessel; or lotion, creams and ointments
- It is also helpful to carry out wet granulation for dry powder
- They are also used in kneading and processing bread dough.

Advantages

- The agitators are lifted easily from the vessel thus cleaning of the bowl is easy
- Less floor space is required for installation

- Material is discharged easily through discharge tube
- Unique movement of both the blades results in fast and efficient mixing of thick material
- It results in quick, intense, homogeneous and dead spot free mixing
- All contact parts are made of stainless steel so no contamination can occur
- It results in faster and better mixing at a lesser time.

Disadvantage

It cannot blend liquid substances.

SILVERSON EMULSIFIER

Silverson emulsifiers are the mixers which are used to change the coarse particles in emulsions and suspensions into fine globules or particles. These emulsifiers create a stable emulsion through finest possible droplet size. The high shear energy introduced into the mix, results in smaller suspended droplets. The high shear rotor/stator design of the Silverson mixer is ideal to produce droplet size of 2 to 5 microns. Finer emulsions down to 0.5 microns can also be obtained, depending on the formulation. Silverson emulsifiers have interchangeable work heads which offer wider functions, such as emulsification, homogenization, disintegration, solubilisation, dispersion, blending, particle size reduction and de-agglomeration. Changing heads also is quick and easy to set. It has a capacity to handle low volumes, nearly 1 ml as well as larger volumes up to 12 litres. These emulsifiers offer excellent reproducibility when scaling up is required. The equipment is found effective for all kind of routine laboratory work, research and development, quality assurance analysis and also for small scale production in industries.

Principle: It works on the principle that the large globules in a coarse emulsion are processed by-passing them under pressure through a narrow orifice so that they are broken into smaller globules.

Construction: It consists of an emulsifier head that contains a number of blades which rotate at high speed which generate a powerful shearing action that is covered with the fine meshed stainless steel sieve. Electric motor fitted at the top is used to rotate the blades. This emulsifier head is placed in the vessel that contains immiscible liquids. As the motor gets start the liquid is sucked through the fine holes and due to the rotation of the blades the oil is reduced into the globules. Exceptionally high shear rates in a four stage mixing/homogenizing process is generated by the machine (Fig. 8.7).

Working: It works in four stages, in a very first stage, the high-speed rotation of the rotor blades within the machine draw liquid and solid materials upwards from the bottom of the vessel and into the centre of the workhead. In stage 2 centrifugal forces then drive the material to the periphery causing mechanical shear. In stage 3, intense hydraulic shear is applied and the product is forced through the stator screen at high velocity. Fresh material is continually drawn into the vessel and particle size is reduced progressively leading to a homogeneous product. In fourth stage, the material expelled from the work head is thrown radially towards the sides of the mixing vessel at high speed. Fresh material is continually drawn into the workhead maintaining the mixing cycle. The horizontal (radial) expulsion and suction into the head generates circulation pattern that minimizes aeration caused by the disturbance of the liquid surface. Emulsifier is widely used for producing emulsions of globule size 2–5 microns.

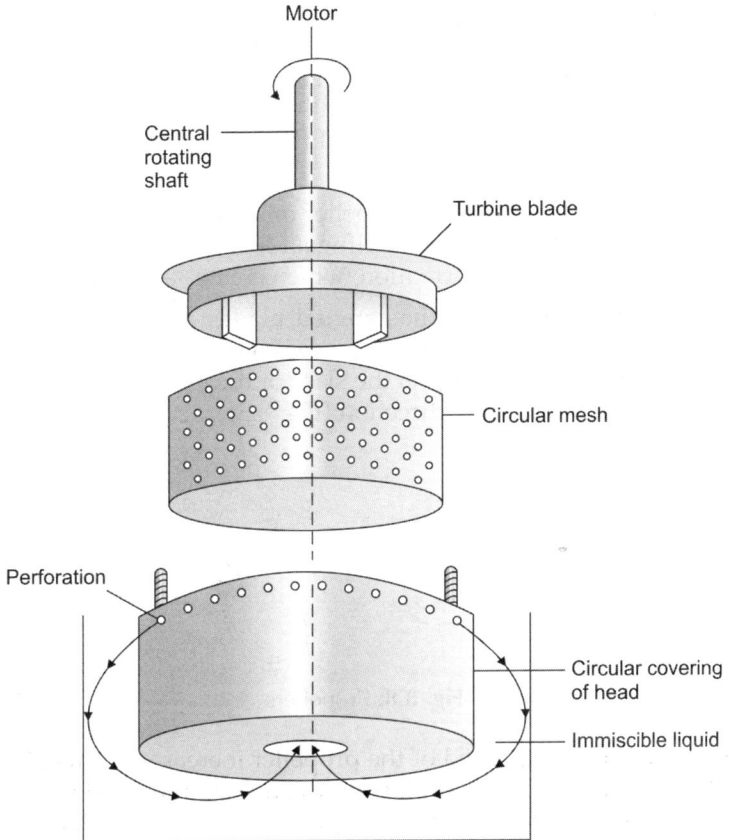

Fig. 8.7: Silverson emulsifier

Advantages

- It helps to get emulsions of range of 0.5 to 5 microns
- It is used for attaining fine suspension both solid and semisolid materials
- It can rapidly disperse gums, alginates, carboxy methyl cellulose, carbopols, etc. resulting in an agglomerate-free solution within 7 minutes due to its high shear action
- In a single operation it can disintegrate animal, vegetable, mineral or synthetic origin matter
- It helps to eliminate problems, such as stratification and rapidly produced a homogeneous product
- It reduces process time compared to other conventional agitators and mixers and thus reduces mixing time up to 90%.

Disadvantages

- High power inputs are required. Also heating of equipment cannot be avoided
- High shear force is imparted which may lead to distortion of the structured compositions.

PROPELLER MIXERS

Propeller mixers are commonly used for medium-scale fluid mixing. The shape of the vessels affects the efficiency of these mixers, e.g. round vessels are better than square ones. Also the proportion of depth of a tank to diameter is also important for functioning of these mixers, for top to bottom blending, the depth should be equal to the diameter of the vessels used. As the depth to diameter decreases, velocity of up-currents generated by propeller mixers gradually reaches to zero, indicating that solid in the material cannot be kept as suspension if the density of solid is greater than the liquid.

Principle: The slant of the blades in propeller mixers causes the fluid to circulate in both radial and axial direction. When centrifugal force is imparted to the liquid by the propeller blades it causes vortex formation, which creates a depression at the shaft.

Construction: A propeller mixer has angled blades generally 3 blade design of stainless-steel for maximum corrosion resistance is most common for liquids and may be right or left handed depending upon the slant of the blades which causes the fluid to circulate in both radial and axial direction (Fig. 8.8).

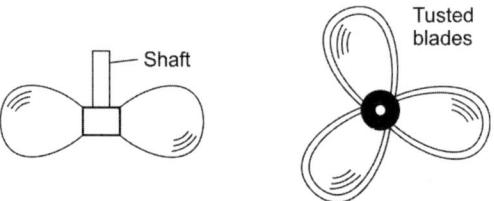

Fig. 8.8: Propellers

Working: As the rotational speed of the propeller increases air may be sucked into the fluid by the formation of a vortex; this may cause frothing and possible oxidation of the components. The problem of air entrapment can be solved by fitting propeller shaft in the vessels in different manners. The problem of the formation of vortex can be suppressed by fitting vertical baffles into the vessel. Vertical baffles divert the rotating fluid from its circular path into the centre of the vessel. The ratio of the diameter of a propeller stirrer to that of the vessel is commonly 1:10–1:20, and it can operate at high speed up to 8000 rpm. The propeller stirrer is not very much efficient to mix the viscous liquids, because they require a fast flow of fluid towards the propeller, which is not possible in viscous liquids.

Applications
- The propeller mixers are used to mix liquids of high viscosity, even of 2000 centipoise viscosity
- These are also preferred for mixing low viscosity emulsions
- The mixers are used for suspensions with particles size up to 0.1 to 0.5 mm maximum, with a drying residue of 10%.

Advantages
- They are used for mixing high volume
- Liquids with maximum viscosity of 2 Pascal/sec or slurry up to 10% solids of fine mesh size can be easily mixed.

Disadvantage
They are not generally effective with liquids of viscosity greater than 5 Pascal/sec, such as glycerine, castor oil, etc.

TURBINE MIXERS

These are the mixers which are used to mix two components fast by attaching the mixer to any variable speed. They are also called pan mixers.

Principle: Turbine mixers with flat blade turbines produce tangential and radial flow but as the speed increases, radial flow is pronounced. In radial flow, the impellers impinge on the vessel walls where it splits into streams. These streams cause mixing by their energy. The pitched blade turbine produces axial flow.

Construction: A turbine consists of a circular disc to which a number of curved blades or short straight blades surrounded by perforated inner and outer diffuser rings are attached. They are used to mix more viscous fluids. These mixers rotate at a lower speed than the propellers (50–200 rpm). They produce constant quality of the mixed material. The mixer is made of stainless steel and gives high returns. All turbine mixers may be fitted with the customer's preferred motor and gearbox or with special drives to comply with (Fig. 8.9).

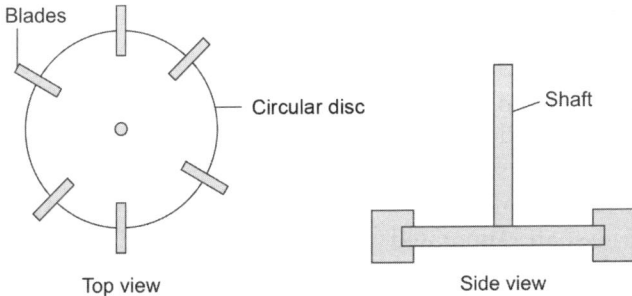

Fig. 8.9: Turbine assembly with blade disc

Working: Turbine mixers are operated in a vessel, while rotating, impeller draws the liquid into the mixer 'head' and forcefully, with radial velocity, pushes the liquid through the perforations, thus overcoming the viscous drag of the bulk of the fluid. A large shear force is produced, when the liquid is forced through the small orifices of the diffuser rings (stationary perforated ring surrounding the turbine). Diffuser ring increases the shear forces therefore, liquid passes through the perforations reducing rotational swirling and vortexing. Turbine mixers are not suitable for the mixing of liquids of very high viscosity, because the material will not be drawn into the mixer head. During operation, air enters into the mixture yielding the bubbles in the material which are not desired.

Applications

- They are available for top and side entry applications for a wide range of mixing applications, such as those found in the asphalt, edible oil, distillery and food industries
- These mixers perform equally well on large and small batches
- Slurries with up to 60% solids, solids of particle size of 10 mesh and liquids of viscosity up to 7000000 centipoise are handled easily with these mixers.

Advantages

- Turbine mixers are user friendly and give better shearing forces than propellers therefore, they are mostly suitable for emulsification

- They are found to be very effective for high viscous solutions with a range of viscosities up to 7 Pascal/second
- If the tank is baffled, they are suitable for large volume liquids with high viscosity
- In low viscous materials of large volumes, turbine creates strong currents which spread throughout the tank destroying immobile pockets. They can handle slurries with 60% solids.

Disadvantage

Degasing is required to remove air bubbles otherwise frothing can occur.

PADDLE MIXERS

Paddle mixers are a type of agitators used in blending, mixing and preparing of dry friable materials, slurries and sludge. These mixers are constructed around a parallel rotating axis with wide-ranging shearing paddles.

Principle: In paddle mixers, the rotating paddles split the mass of the material while blending thus generating convection movement in the vessel which leads to thorough mixing. Also, due to position of paddles at an angle, the mixer shows an excellent axial and radial dispersion which aids in mixing. If additional accessories, such as choppers are placed, the additional energy is created which is used to break lumps or agglomerates in the dispersion.

Construction: Paddle mixer consists of paddles mounted on twin shafts in a 'W' shaped trough. The shaft is operated at a specific speed and an overlapping motion is created by the paddles. Such a synchronized effect of shaft and paddle leads to rapid fluidization and ensures excellent transport of particles within the W-shaped vessel. This type of mixer was patented by the Norwegian inventor Halvor Forberg and is also popularly known as the Forberg fluidized zone mixer. The material generally occupies 25% of the total volume of the trough that is; it is slightly above the shafts. The material to be mixed is charged from the top of the trough. Liquid spraying arrangement is also possible if required. The head space is sufficient to provide air around the particles so that they can move freely. The peripheral speed of the paddles is approximately 100 metres per minute which ensures thorough mixing. Discharge of the mixed material is through the two large doors located at the bottom of the vessel. Discharge valves, such as half bomb bay doors, spherical disc valves can also be placed (Fig. 8.10).

Working: They have the same procedure as ribbon mixers, i.e. they are usually housed in a semi-cylinder type, but instead of ribbon shapes, these mixers have paddle-shaped blades extended from the axis. In this type of mixers a number of paddles consist of a central hub which is attached to a vertical shaft with long flat blades attached to it vertically and are rotated with a low speed of around 100 rpm. Two or four blades are common. For mixing the liquids, with low viscosity simple flat paddles are used, which

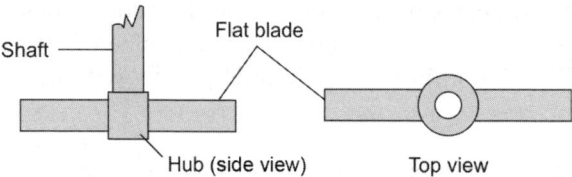

Fig. 8.10: Paddle type of agitator

push the liquid radially and tangentially with almost no axial action unless blades are pitched. In deep tanks several paddles are attached one above the other on the same shaft. For the mixing of highly viscous fluid, mixers are attached with number of blades, shaped to fit closely to the surface of the vessel to avoid the dead spot and deposited solids. An alternative, planetary motion mixer is also in existence to mix the highly viscous liquids, which consists of small paddles, that rotates on its own axis. A variety of paddle mixers are available with different size and shape, which depends upon the character and viscosity of the liquid that has to be mixed.

Applications
- Paddles are used for the manufacturing of antidiarrheal mixtures, e.g. bismuth-kaolin, antacid suspensions, agar and pectin related purgatives
- Paddle mixers are often used for mixing heavy solids, slurry mixing, wet-dry mixing and mixing of other high viscosity liquid, such as sludge and fertilizers
- They are used frequently for mixing dry constituents, such as coffee, sugar, minerals, chemicals and agricultural feed among many other food, pharmaceutical and chemical products.

Advantages
- Due to low speed mixing, formation of vortex is not possible with paddle impellers
- Mixing homogeneity of 98–99% can be achieved using twin shaft paddle mixer.

Disadvantage
As mixing of the suspension with paddles is poor therefore, baffled tanks are required.

VERY SHORT ANSWER QUESTIONS

1. Name and explain the principle of the equipment used for semisolid mixing.
2. What is mixing? Enlist the equipment used in pharma industries.
3. Differentiate with suitable example between mixing and agitation.
4. Giving suitable example of liquids based on their miscibility.
5. Name and give advantages for a equipment used for semisolids mixing.

SHORT ANSWER QUESTIONS

1. What are factors affecting mixing?
2. Give a detail note on classification of mixtures.
3. How is convective mixing different from diffusive mixing?
4. What is the difference between propeller and turbines?
5. What do you understand by bulk transport?
6. Give two advantages of Silverson emulsifier.

LONG ANSWER QUESTIONS

1. Discuss the advantages and disadvantages of sigma blender.

2. Explain the construction and working of planetary mixer.

3. What are the advantages and disadvantages of Ribbon blenders?

4. Explain the working of a mixer for semisolid material.

5. Discuss the principle, working and advantages of double cone blender.

6. Discuss principles, construction, working, uses, merits and demerits of propellers and turbines.

7. Give a detail note on twin shell blender.

MULTIPLE CHOICE QUESTIONS

1. Helical screw agitator is used for ....
   a. Mixing highly viscous paste
   b. Blending immiscible liquid
   c. Mixing liquids at very high temperature
   d. Mixing solids

2. Mixing index is applicable for mixing of solids at zero time.
   a. True   b. False

3. Which of the following conditions show that a certain industrial mixer is the best?
   a. Power load for mixing is minimum
   b. Standard deviation is minimum
   c. Time required for mixing is minimum
   d. All of above

4. A propeller agitator ....
   a. Produces mainly axial flow   b. Used for mixing high viscous pastes
   c. Runs at slow speed   d. Used for low viscous fluids

5. Highly viscous liquids and pastes, are agitated by ....
   a. Propellers   b. Turbine agitators
   c. Multiple blade paddles   d. Blenders

6. Factors affecting mixing are:
   a. Particle shape   b. Size
   c. Both   d. None

7. Which of the following with respect to mixing is true?
   a. It is used to distribute heat uniformly to all the components of the mixture
   b. Mixing becomes difficult when one of the phases to be mixed is in minor quantity
   c. Solid-solid mixing is more difficult than other phase
   d. All of the above

8. **Rate of mixing at any time is given by the extent of mixing at that particular time.**
   a. True   b. False

9. **The force used for mixing by mixing equipment for pastes and dough is** ....
   a. Centrifugal smearing   b. Impact
   c. Tumbling   d. All of the above

10. **Statement 1: Effectiveness of mixing in kneaders depends on the blade design. Statement 2: Kneaders have a high clearance between the two oppositely rotating blades and the vessel.**
    a. True, False   b. True, True
    c. False, False   d. False, True

11. **Statement 1: Which mixture is used when one of the components is very less in quantity? Statement 2: This mixer is used to mix items in savory or a snack item.**
    a. Ribbon mixer, planetary mixer
    b. Planetary mixer, double cone mixer
    c. Double cone mixer, double cone mixer
    d. Planetary mixer, planetary mixer

12. **The clearance between the impeller and the vessel in a mixer is usually kept** ....
    a. High   b. Low
    c. Cannot be determined   d. None of the mentioned

13. **Statement 1: Kneaders are specially used for pastry/viscous liquids in the food industry. Statement 2: Kneaders are used for mixing dough with fats and making them homogeneous mixtures.**
    a. True, False   b. True, True
    c. False, False   d. False, True

Filtration

Iram Khan and Manju Sharma

Filtration may be defined as the process of separating the solids from a fluid by means of a porous medium that allows the fluid to pass through it but retain the solid materials. The term fluid may include liquids as well as gases.

Slurry, the suspension of solid and liquid that is to be filtered is known as slurry. *The filter medium* is *the porous medium* that filters the suspension and the accumulated solid matter is known as *filter cake*. The clear liquid that is passed through the filter medium is known as *filtrate*.

OBJECTIVES

- To eliminate the dispersing fluid and recover solid particles
- To recover dispersing fluid by eliminating the contaminant particles.

APPLICATIONS

- It is used for separation of particles and fluid in a suspension or emulsion pharmaceutical preparations to obtain a clear solution as it is more acceptable to patients
- It is used for production of sterile products by use of (HEPA) filters (or) laminar air bench that helps in providing sterile environment during manufacture of sterile products
- For filtration of thermo labile substances in which heat sterilization is not applicable bacteria proof filters can be used
- It is used for production of bulk drugs where filtration is a necessary step for the removal of impurities from the products
- It is used in manufacturing of liquid orals and for obtaining clear solutions in which removal of foreign impurities is necessary, e.g. eyedrops, aromatic water preparations, syrups, elixirs
- It can also be used with other unit operations to process the feed stream such as biofilter, i.e. a combination of filter and a biological digestion device
- It is also helpful in effluent and waste water treatment.

THEORY OF FILTRATION

The mechanisms in which the solid particles are retained on the filter medium have some significance only in the early stage of filtration process. As once a primary layer of particles gets deposited on the medium, then the process of filtration is affected only by the filter cake. The exact mechanism of filtration has greater importance in the process of clarification, where the proportion of solid is very low. Following are some mechanisms:

Entanglement

In this mechanism filter medium consists of cloth or porous belt in which particles become entangled in the fibres. Usually, the particles are smaller than the pores.

Straining

In this type of filtration process solid particles are retained in the filter medium due to larger particles than the pore size of filter medium.

Impingement

In this process solid particles move along the path of streamline flow of liquid and the filter medium and are retained on the filter.

Attractive Forces

Solid particle may be deposited on the filter due to attractive forces between particles and filter medium, e.g. electrostatic precipitation.

Rate of Filtration

The main objective of the filtration process is to filter the slurry as fast as possible. The rate of filtration was first studied by Darcy in 1830. The equation that correlates the rate of filtration and affecting factors are known a *Darcy's law*, which can be expressed as follows:

$$dv/dt = KA\Delta P/\eta L$$

where,

dv/dt = Rate of filtration

K = Constant for the filter medium and filter cake

A = Area of filter medium

ΔP = Pressure drop across the filter cake and filter medium

L = Thickness of the filter cake

η = Viscosity of filtrate

Poiseuille's Equation

According to Poiseuille's law, filtration is similar to the streamline flow of a liquid under pressure through capillaries. When the filter cake is composed of a bulk mass of particles, the rate of filtration is expressed by Poiseuille's equation.

Poiseuille's equation may be expressed as:

$$dv/dt = \Delta P\pi r^4/8\eta l$$

where,

dv/dt = Rate of filtration

r = Radius of the capillary in the filter bed

ΔP = Pressure drop across the filter cake and filter medium

l = Thickness of the filter cake

η = Viscosity of filtrate

Kozeny-Carman Equation

The compressibility of the cake has a greater effect on the flow rate of liquids, because flow rate is proportional to $\varepsilon^3/(1-\varepsilon)^2$. Kozeny-Carman equation can be expressed by following equation:

$$dv/dt = A\Delta P\varepsilon^3/\eta S^2 K(1-\varepsilon)^2$$

ε = Porosity of the cake

S = Specific surface area of the particles comprising the cake

K = Constant (usually taken as 5)

FILTER MEDIA

Filter medium act as a support for the filter cake and it is also responsible for the retention of the solids. Filter medium must have sufficient mechanical strength, should be inert, have low resistance to flow and should not absorb the dissolved material. The magnitude of the resistance of the filter medium will change due to the deposition of solid, which may block the pores or may form bridge over the entrances of the capillaries. So, to avoid the blocked pores, the pressure should be kept low at the beginning. The material that may be used as filter medium includes:

- Woven material such as cloth or felt, which is made up of cotton, wool, glass, silk, metal or rayon and nylon, etc. The choice of the fibre depends on the chemical nature of the slurry
- Perforated metal sheet, e.g. stainless steel plates, may also be used as filter medium
- Pre-fabricated single unit porous solids are more convenient and effective filter medium, e.g. sintered glass, single metal, porous plastics, earthware filters
- Bed of granular solid built-up on a supportive medium. The sizes of solids are chosen according to the needs of the process. Typical examples of solids that are used for this purpose are sand, paper pulp, asbestos, kieselguhr and gravel.

FILTER AIDS

The main purpose of the use of filter aids is to prevent the medium from becoming blocked and to form an open porous cake to reduce the resistance of the filter cake or filter medium against the flow of filtrate. Filter aids are used only for clarification process. The filter aids must be light, porous, inert solid and should have adsorptive properties that can remove solids from the filtrate.

It may be used by two ways:

a. By forming a coat over the filter medium by filtering a suspension of filter aids that can coat the medium up to 0.5 kg/m³.

b. Filter aids may be used adding it to the slurry up to 0.1 to 0.5% kieselguhr, talc, bentonite, and paper pulp, charcoal are the main examples of the filter aids.

FACTORS AFFECTING FILTRATION

Some of the factors that may affect the rate of filtration include:

- The properties of liquids, e.g. viscosity, density, corrosiveness, etc.
- The properties of the solids, e.g. particle size, particle shape, rigidity, compressibility, particles size distribution, etc.
- Ratio of solid and liquid in the study
- Temperature of the suspension.

Properties of the Filter Medium and Filter Cake

The resistance of the filter medium and filter cake is of significance on the laboratory scale. The magnitude of the resistance will change due to the early layers of solids which may block the pores may form bridges over the entrances to the channels. The resistance of the cake is affected by a number of fundamental properties of the solids that includes surface area of the particles and it is also observed that rate of filtration is increased with the decrease in the resistance of the filter cake.

Area of the Filter Medium

The rate of the filtration can be increased by making use of large area filters because the total volume of filtrate is proportional to the area of filter.

Pressure Drop Across the Filter Medium

The rate of filtration is directly proportional to the pressure drop across the filter medium and filter cake. The pressure drop can be achieved by number of ways:

Gravity: A pressure difference can be achieved by maintaining the filter medium above a head of slurry. The developed pressure will depend on the density of the suspension.

Reduced pressure: The pressure difference across the filter can be created by a vacuum pump via connecting the filtrate receiver. The magnitude of the pressure will be below the atmospheric pressure. Reduction of pressure may lower the boiling point of the liquid that causes the possibility of the filtrate to boil in the receiver.

Pressure: Suitable pressure difference across the filter medium can be obtained by applying pressure to the surface of the slurry. The pressure difference obtained by this method will be greater than reduced method.

Viscosity of the filtrate: The viscosity of the liquid, not the slurry, has the greater influence on the filtration rate of the suspension. The resistance to flow increases with increase in the viscosity of the filtrate. Hence, the rate of filtration is inversely proportional to the viscosity of the liquid. The rate of filtration may be increased by increasing the temperature of the liquid that lowers the viscosity of the liquid, but increase in temperature is not suitable for thermo labile substances.

Thickness of Filter Cake

The rate of filtration is inversely proportional to the thickness of filter cake. The cake thickness will be affected by area of filtration. So, by increasing the area of filtration, we can increase the filtration rate because it will reduce the thickness of filter cake. The reduction in the thickness of filter cake may also be done by preliminary decantation or straining process, which will lower the solid content of the slurry.

Filters: The equipment used for the process of filtration are known as filters that acts as a tool in separation processes for solids and liquids.

They are Classified as

- **On the basis of application of external force:**
  - *Pressure filters*, e.g. plate and frame filter press and metafilter
  - *Vacuum filters*, e.g. filter leaf
  - Centrifugal filters.

- **On the basis of the operation of the filtration:**
  - *Continuous filtration*: Filtrate and discharge gets separated steadily and uninterrupted
  - *Discontinuous filtration*: Filtrate is removed continuously and discharge of filtered solids is intermittent.
- **On the basis of the nature of filtration:**
  - *Cake filters*: Involves removal of large amounts of solids (crystals)
  - *Clarification filters*: Involves removal of small amounts of solids
  - *Cross-flow filters*: At a fairly high velocity across the filter medium feed of suspension flows under pressure.
- **On the basis of scaling up:**
  - *Batch filtration (small scale)*: It includes parameters to be controlled are pressure drop, concentration of slurry.
  - *Continuous filtration (large scale)*: The parameters to be controlled is pressure drop, concentration of slurry, drum speed.

  Filter leaf: It is a simplest form of filter.

  Principle: It consists of a longitudinal drainage screen covered with a filter cloth. The mechanism is surface filtration and acts as a sieve or strainer. By applying pressure or vacuum rate of filtration can be increased.

  Construction: It consists of a frame with a drainage screen or grooved plate and the whole unit is covered with a filter cloth (Fig. 9.1). The frame may be of any shape like square, rectangular or circular. Filtering area can be alter by employing a suitable

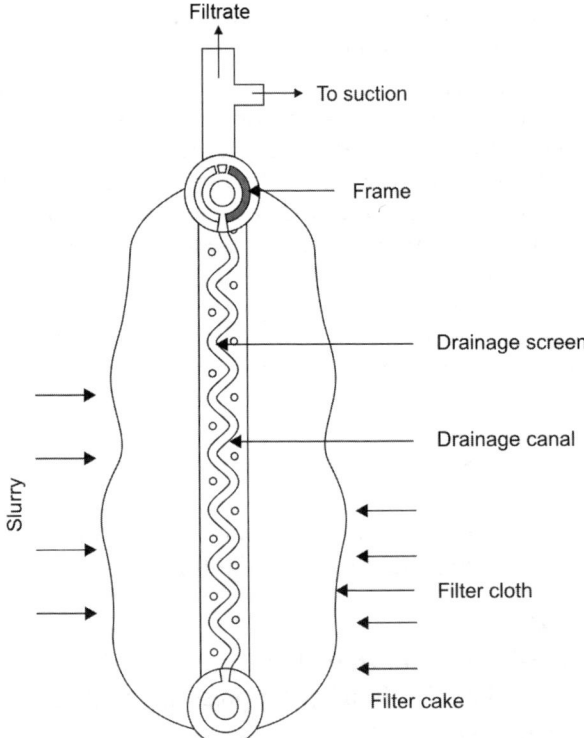

Fig. 9.1: Filter leaf

number of filter units and by using suitable vessels, the pressure difference maintained by vacuum or by applying pressure up to the 8 bars. The leaf filters are most suitable if the solid content in the slurry is up to 5%. Washing efficiency is comparatively very high in the leaf filters.

Working: The filter leaf is immersed in the slurry and vacuum system and a receiver is connected to the outlet. By using this method, slurry can be filtered from any vessel and by dipping the leaf in a vessel of water the cake can be easily washed. The cake can be easily removed by using reverse air flow. Filtration process can be performed by enclosing the filter leaf in a specific vessel into which the slurry is pumped under pressure. This process is generally used, when a number of leaves are joined to a common outlet, in order to offer a large filtration area.

Uses

It is used for the slurry containing solid content not above 5%, i.e dilute suspensions.

Advantages

- From any vessel the slurry can be filtered
- The cake can be simply washed by immersing the filter in a water vessel
- Removal of the cake is easily done by the use of reverse air flow
- It can be modified by connecting number of units
- Labour costs not too high.

Disadvantages

- If the cake is heavy and thick it becomes difficult to hold the pressure on the leaf
- Precoating is done to avoid retention of cake and is not a simple operation
- Large space and high maintenance required.

ROTARY FILTER

Principle: Rotary filter is continuous in operation. It consists of a system that can remove the filter cake. So, they are suitable for filtering the concentrated slurry. They filter the slurry under vacuum through sieve-like mechanism on a rotating drum surface.

Construction: Rotary drum filter consists of a metal cylinder that is mounted horizontally (Fig. 9.2). The rotary drum is up to 3 meter in diameter and 3.5 meter in length, having an area of 20 meter square. The curved surface is perforated which supports filter cloth of the rotary filter. The drum is radically divided into separated compartments. By an internal pipe each compartment is connected to the centre of the drum through a rotating valve.

Working: During operation drum rotates at low speed. The drum just enters the slurry in the trough. When it (drum) dips in the slurry, due to the applied vacuum, the solid is deposited on the drum surface. The liquid filtered through the cloth and enter in an internal pipe and valve and at last it is collected in collecting tank.

After leaving the slurry section, drum enters the drainage area. Special attachment, like, cake compression rollers, may be included at this section. By this attachment, cake is consolidated by the compression mechanism. This process improves the efficiency of the washing and drying process. From the drainage section, the drum enters the water wash area. In this section water is poured on the cake. In order to suck the water wash and air through the solid cake, a separate vacuum system is

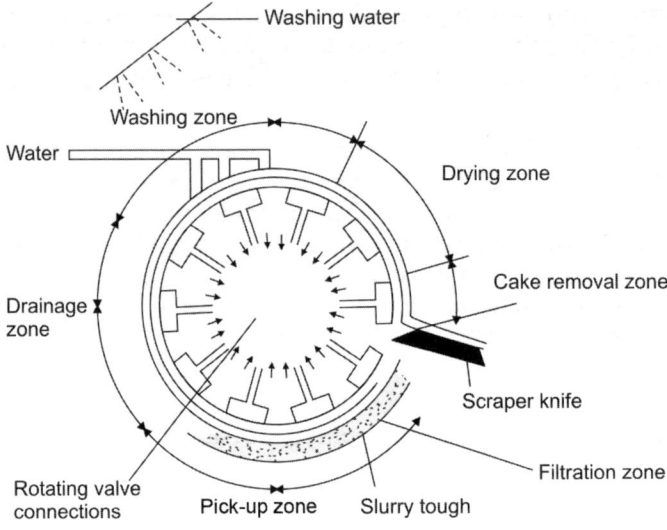

Fig. 9.2: Rotary drum filter

applied. Wash water is filtered into a separate collecting tank. After, leaving washing zone, drum enters into the drying zone where hot air is blown on the cake. Finally, the cake is scraped by knife and then drum is ready to complete another revolution.

Uses
- It is used for large quantities of slurry
- It is suitable for slurry containing considerable amounts of solids in the range of 15–30%.

Advantages
- Filtration area is large
- It is a continuous process and a complete automatic process
- The labour costs are very low
- Thickness of cake on the drum can be controlled by varying the speed of drum.

Disadvantages
- The rotary filter is very expensive process and its functioning is very complex
- Due to the air drawn through by the vacuum system the cake may break
- The pressure difference should not be more than 1 bar.

META FILTER (EDGE FILTER)

Principle: Meta filters are used as a surface filtration unit for coarse particles. It contains metal rings having semicircular projections which are arranged as a nest to form channels on the edge that offers resistance to the flow of solids.

Construction: Meta filter consists of a series of metal rings (Figs 9.3A and B). The thickness of the ring is about 0.8 mm and inner as well as outer diameters are about 15 and 22 mm respectively. These rings are threaded to formed channel on the edges. Each metal rings has various semicircular projections on one side of the surface. These projections are arranged the same way up. The rings are tightened on the drainage rod with nut. Hence also known as edge filters. These filters are mounted in a vessels

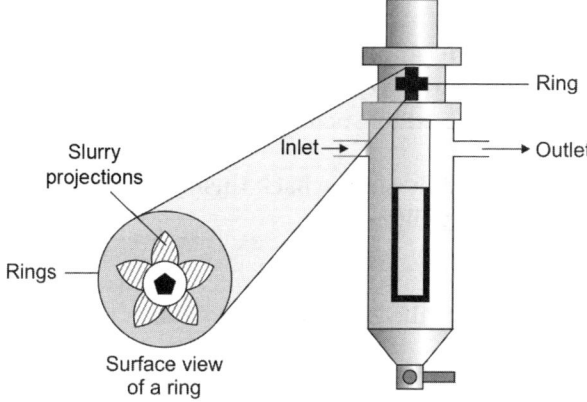

Fig. 9.3A: An edge filter

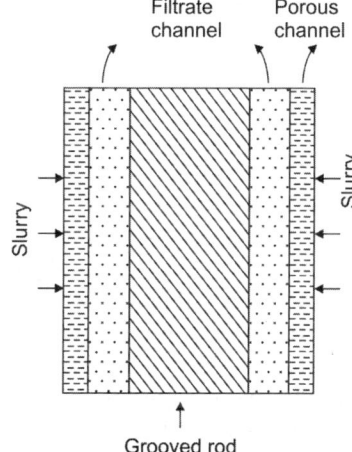

Fig. 9.3B: Mechanism of filtration through metafilters

and may be operated by the application of reduced pressure to the outlet direction or by pumping the slurry under pressure. To separate the fine particles from the slurry, first, a bed of a suitable material (e.g. kieselguhr) is built-up.

Working: In it filters are placed in a vessel and operated by pumping the slurry under pressure or occasionally by the applications of reduced pressure to the outlet side. Then the slurry passes through the channels formed on the edge between the rings and the clear liquid rises up and gets collected from the outlet into the receiver. It works as a strainer. To separate fine particles a bed of kieselguhr is first built-up. The pack of the rings works as a base on which a true filter medium can be supported.

Uses

- It is used for syrups clarification
- It is mainly used for filtering of injections
- It can be used for viscous liquids
- Meta filter are mostly used for insulin liquors.

Advantages

- Edge filter can be used under high pressure
- Running cost is very low and is very economical process
- They can be easily constructed by such metal that can provide excellent resistance against corrosion
- Cake can be easily removed by simple back flushing with water
- Sterile product can be easily filtered.

Disadvantages

The small surface area restricts the collection of solids.

FILTER PRESS

Principle: A **filter press** is used in separation processes, specifically in solid/liquid separation using pressure based principle provided by a slurry pump. It is used in fixed-volume and batch operations, therefore, the operation must be stopped to discharge the filter cake before the next batch can be started. The major components are the skeleton and the filter pack. The skeleton holds the filter pack together while pressure is being developed inside the filtration chamber. The chamber can only hold a specific volume of solids.

Construction: Plate and frame filter is made up of two types of units known as plate and frame. Filter medium usually filter cloth is placed between plate and frames as shown in Fig. 9.4. It may be made by various types of metal to prevent corrosion or metal contamination of the product. Non-metals generally plastic and wood are also used as satisfactory material of construction. There are many types of filter presses. The simplest type is open delivery system. It consists of single conduit for introduction of the slurry and the wash and a single opening in each plate for removal of the liquid. Other is closed delivery system. It consists of separate conduits for introducing the slurry and wash water. Some also have separate conduit for removing filtrate and wash water. The conduit may be at the corner, at the centre or at intermediate location. Plate has a studded or grooved surface to support the filter cloth and an outlet for the filtrate.

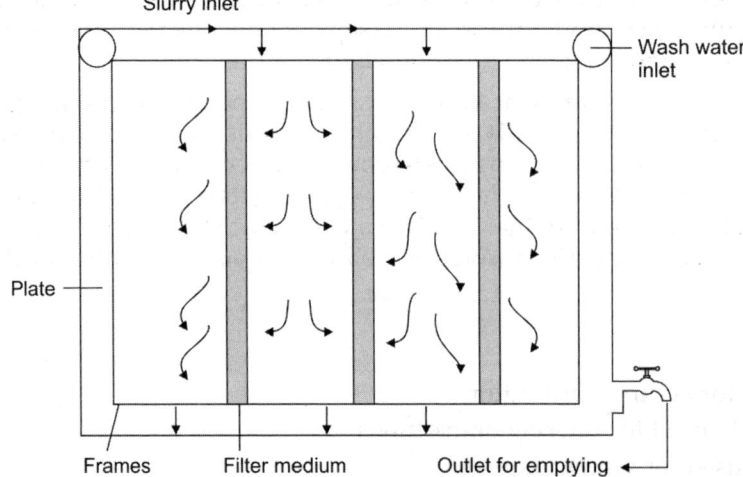

Fig. 9.4: Plate and frame filter press

Working: From the feed channel slurry enters the frame and the filtrate passes through the filter medium on the surface of the plate. The filter cake is formed of solid from the slurry in the frame. The thickness of the cake can be changed by using frame of different thickness. Depending on the resistance of the filter cake and solids mass of the slurry, there will be a possible thickness of filter cake for any slurry. As the filtration continues, the rate of filtration decreases due to increase in resistance of the cake.

The filtrate flows down to the surface of the plate and comes through the outlet. Filtration is continued till the frame is full with the filter cake. The process is terminated due to the thickness of cake, the frame emptied, channels of the plates and frames, these joining together to form a channel.

Washing of plate and frame filters: The ordinary plate and frame press is not suitable to wash the filter cake. During the filtration process in filter press, two cake are build in frame, melting eventually in the middle.

So, to wash the filter cake, a modified plate and frame press is used. In this press special plate and frame are used which have an additional channel to carry wash water. In this type of press half of the plate are connected with wash water channel to the surface of the plates and these special plates are marked by three dots. The sequence of arrangement of plate and frame can be separated by dots.

Filtration proceeds till the frames are filled with cake and to wash the filter cake the outlets on the washing plates are closed. Then washed water is pumped into the washing channel and the water enters the inlets of the washing plates. Water passes and enters into frame which contain the cake that needs to wash through the filter cloth and enters the plate down the surface. Finally water escapes from the outlet on the plate. It is necessary to allow the frame to fill completely with the cake as it would facilitate correct washing of the cake.

Uses

Plate and frame presses are widely used, when the cake is valuable and relatively small in quantity.

Advantages

- It has a large filtering area as compared to a small floor space
- Efficient washing of cake is possible
- It is simple to construct and a wide variety of materials can be used, e.g. cast iron, bronze, stainless steel, wood, plastic, etc.
- Operation and maintenance is simple
- It produces dry cake.

Disadvantages

- It is an expensive process
- It is used for slurries containing less than about 5% solids
- It is a batch process, so time consuming and non productive.

MEMBRANE FILTERS

Principle: They act like a sieve trapping particulate matter on their surface. It performs separations by retaining particles larger than its pore size on the surface of the membrane. Particles with a diameter below the rated pore size may either pass through the membrane or get within the membrane.

Construction: It mainly consists of cellulose acetate, cellulose nitrates, polytetrafluoroethylene (PTFE), polyvinylchloride, nylon, etc. having the shape of discs or cartridges. Membrane filter holders accept membranes from 13 to 293 mm in diameter. Several grades of filters are available with pore sizes ranging from 0.010 ± 0.002 to 5.0 ± 1.2 micron. During use membrane filters are supported on a rigid base of perforated metal, plastic or coarse sintered glass as in the case of fibrous pad filter (Fig. 9.5).

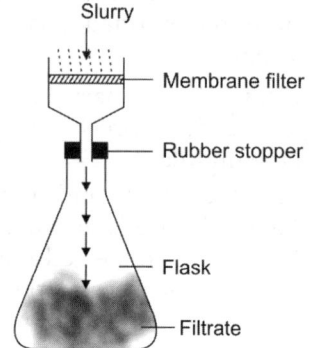

Fig. 9.5: Membrane filters assembly

Working: The membrane filter is fitted in the filter holder and soaked in water. From filtrate side or by pressing through positive pressure from the slurry side the slurry can be drawn through the membrane under vacuum. If the solution to be filtered contains a considerable quantity of suspended matter, preliminary filtration through a suitable depth filter avoids clogging of the membrane filter. They are brittle when dry and can be stored indefinitely in the dry state but are fairly tough when wet.

Uses

- It is used in aerosol
- It is also applicable in radioactivity
- Mainly used for particle sizing.

Advantages

- During prolonged filtration no bacterial growth through the filter takes place
- They are disposable and no cross contamination take place
- They yield no fibres or alkali into the filtrate hence adsorption is negligible
- Filtration rate is high.

Disadvantages

- It shows clogging
- Less resistant to solvents like chloroform.

CARTRIDGE FILTERS

Cartridge filters are the machines which is used in filtration purpose, by using the filtration technology of removing solid matter and suspended impurities from a fluid stream by passing it through a variety of microporous filters, ultrafiltration units, green sand cartridge filters, activated carbon cartridge filters, diatomaceous earth and multimedia cartridge filters. Cartridge filters use a variety of media to remove contaminants, depending on your application. The filter media in our cartridge filters encompass a wide range from sand, anthracite and quartz to conditioned media for iron and manganese removal, and activated carbon. Cartridge filters range in style from particulate and high purity water cartridge filters, to activated carbon filters, vent cartridge filters and replacement cartridge filters for laboratory usage. Our cartridge filters are available in a wide variety of sizes, capabilities, and specific end caps. Cartridge filters have a filtration rate from 0.1 up to 500 micron. They are manufactured by affixing the fabric or polymer to a central core and they are usually rigid or semirigid. Cartridge filters are disposable and easily replaceable (Table 9.1).

Principle: The filtration action is done mainly by sieve like action and the particles retained on the surface. It is a thin porous membrane containing pre-filter and membrane filter in a single unit.

Construction: It consists of cylindrical configuration made with disposable or changeable filter media. They are made of either plastic or metal. It consists of two membrane filters (sieve like) made of polypropylene a prefilter and an actual filter used for filtration surrounded by protective layer as shown in Fig. 9.6. The cartridges are housed in a holder and numbers of them are placed in same housing. The housing is closed with a lid and has provisions for slurry inlet and filtrate outlet.

The cartridge filter systems are basically of two kinds:

1. *Smaller systems*: They are usually used as a single wound cartridge also used in a home filtering system usually constructed of body made-up of plastic or stainless steel. The lid contains the outlet ports, inlet ports and pressure relief valve. Taps or ports for pressure gauges are containing in smaller cartridge filter systems.
2. Larger systems usually consist of multiple cartridge filters can be used either pleated or wound filters.

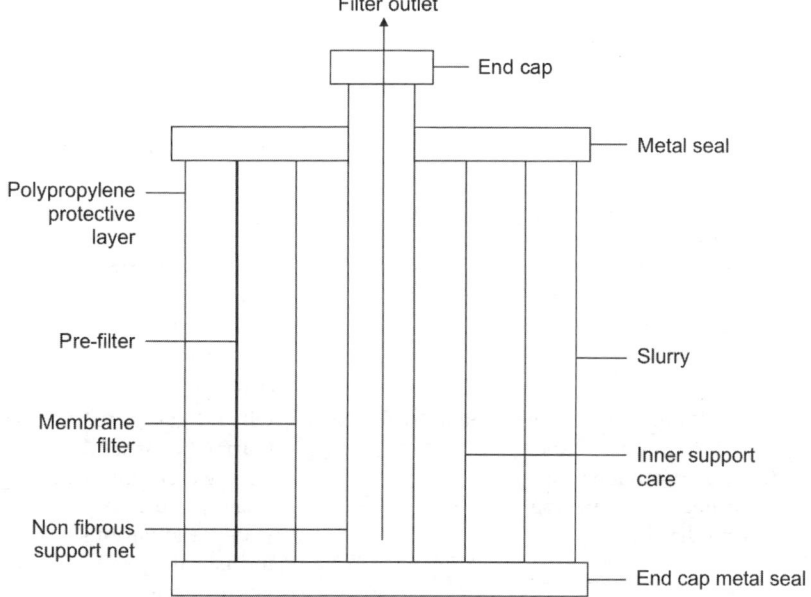

Fig. 9.6: Cartridge filter

Table 9.1: Description of the cartridge filter

Types of filters	Material	Filtration	Applications	Filtration range (micron)
Wound cartridge filters	Natural or synthetic yards, which are wounded around a central tube or former	Sand, scale, lime, rust, fine particles.	Drinking water, boilers, washing machines, pre-filtration in water treatment, sea water desalination, process water, chemical processes.	0.5–150
Melt-blown cartridge filters	One-pieces cordless construction, consisting of pure polypropylene micro fibers, thermally bonded to prevent any fiber migration.	Sand, scale, lime, rust, fine particles	Water treatment, pure water pre-filtration, fine chemicals, reverse osmosis, sea water desalination, beverages, solvents, cosmetics.	1–75
Activated carbon cartridge filters	Polypropylene fleece and net, or washed machines, anti-chlorine polypropylene yarn and activated granular carbon.	Removal of taste contamination, pesticides and organic substances treatment in nourishing, pre-treatment for reverse osmosis plants, pharma-ceutical and chemical plants	Potable water, washing machines, anti-chlorine treatment in alimentary, chemical and pharma-ceutical industry, pre-treatment for reverse osmosis units	1–25
Stainless steel cartridge filters	Stainless steel cartridge filter of inner core of polypropylene	Sand and rust	Drinking water, in washing machines, in boilers, pre-filtration process of pumps, in irrigation and also in protecting industrial systems	70
Pleated cartridge filters	Pleated polypropylene or stainless steel filtering net of stainless steel having a inner core of polypropylene	Sand and rust	Drinking water, boilers, washing machines, pre-filtration of water pumps, irrigation systems, protection of industrial fittings.	50
Oil-block cartridge filters	Polypropylene caps and outer shell and polypropylene caps filled by absorption media	Sand, scales, rust	Oil and gas industry, marine ballast and bilge water treatment systems, surface water, and various industrial applications	40

Working: The slurry is pumped into the catridge holder and passes through catridge filter unit by the mechanism of straining. The clear liquid passes to the center and moves up and gets collected through the outlet.

Uses

- It is useful for the preparation of the particulate free solutions for the parenteral and ophthalmic uses
- They have application in a water treatment plant for surface water treatment rule compliance, prefiltration prior to subsequent treatment and in solids removal.

Advantages

- It can be used for sterile products
- Catridges are self-cleaning
- Reusing and rapid disassembling of the filter media
- Catridge do not become brittle when dry
- They reduce handling of solutions as they are used in line continuous filtration
- Less contamination.

Disadvantages

- Costly and difficult for cleaning
- The components provide by manufacturers are generally not interchangeable.

SEITZ FILTER

Principle: The filtration occurs through pad or sheet ranging from 2 mm thickness to desired size range. It follows the mechanism similar to depth filtration.

Construction: It consists of two parts: Lower part fitted with a perforated plate over which compressed asbestos pad is placed. Upper part has a value through which pressure can be applied. Both parts joined together by winged nuts (Fig. 9.7).

Working: It consists of perforated discs and asbestos sheet which is made-up of asbestos fibers but may also contain cellulose and alkaline earth metals. In this process slurry penetrates to a point where the diameter of solid particles is greater than that of

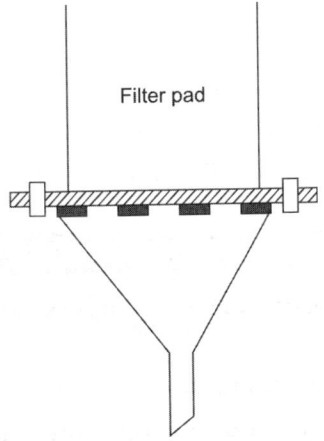

Filter pad

Fig. 9.7: Seitz filter

the tortuous void or channel. The solid gets retained by physical restriction or even by adsorption properties of the medium.

Applications

It is used for air filtration.

Advantages

- No risk of contaminating the filtrate
- Apparatus is very simple to use
- For viscous solution they are more suitable.

Disadvantages

- Asbestos may shed loose fibres
- Pad may absorb sufficient amount of medicament
- They are fragile.

VERY SHORT QUESTIONS

1. What is filtration? Explain its objectives.
2. Define filter aids. List its properties.
3. What is the mechanism of membrane in filtration?
4. Enlist the advantages of Seitz filter and explain principle.
5. Differentiate between surface and depth filtration?

SHORT QUESTIONS

1. Classify filtration and mention its applications.
2. Give a detail account on mechanism of filtration.
3. Explain the principle, construction, working and uses of membrane filter.
4. Explain the principle, construction, working and uses of filter used for viscous liquids.
5. Explain with reason why:
   a. How back washing is achieved in filtration?
   b. Filter aids improve the rate of filtration.
6. Differentiate between vacuum filter and membrane filter.

LONG QUESTIONS

1. Explain the principle, construction, working, uses, advantages and disadvantages of filter leaf.
2. State the factors affecting filtration.
3. Explain the principle, construction, working, uses, advantages and disadvantages of frame filter.

4. Write a detail note on rotary drum filter.

5. Write the principle, construction, working and uses of filter used for clarification of syrups.

6. Write a principle, construction, working and uses of cartridge filter.

MULTIPLE CHOICE QUESTIONS

1. Cloth filter is mainly made of:
   - a. Canvas
   - b. Synthetic fabrics
   - c. Metal or glass fiber
   - d. All of these

2. Process used for separation of insoluble particles from liquids is:
   - a. Drying
   - b. Filtration
   - c. Sieving
   - d. Extraction

3. An axial compressor is said to be .... pressure ratio turbo machine.
   - a. High
   - b. Low
   - c. Medium
   - d. Constant

4. The flow area .... as to density variation from inlet to exit.
   - a. Reduces
   - b. Increases
   - c. Remains same
   - d. Constant

5. In an axial turbine, the kinetic energy of combustion gas is converted to mechanical power by ....
   - a. Shear action
   - b. Axial action
   - c. Impulse action
   - d. Tear action

6. Filter used for continuous mode of filtration is:
   - a. Plate and frame
   - b. Spiral wound
   - c. Rotary vacuum
   - d. Tubular

7. High pressure drop is caused if the aperture size of the filtration medium is too small.
   - a. True
   - b. False

8. Statement 1: Filter cake helps to increase the efficiency of filtration.
   Statement 2: Filter aid is added to the filter cake to obtain the filter cake as the desired product.
   - a. True, False
   - b. True, True
   - c. False, False
   - d. False, True

9. Express the effect of pressure drop on the rate of filtration?
   - a. Increases
   - b. Decreases
   - c. Varies depending on the compressibility
   - d. None of the above

10. **Choose the cheapest filtration equipment.**
    a. Plate and frame filter press
    b. Pressure leaf filter press
    c. Continuous rotary vacuum filter press
    d. None of above

11. **Name the filtration equipment that offers maximum pressure drop.**
    a. Plate and frame filter press
    b. Pressure leaf filter press
    c. Continuous rotary vacuum filter press
    d. None of the above

12. **Out of the following filtration equipment which operates under continuous operation.**
    a. Plate and frame filter press
    b. Pressure leaf filter press
    c. Continuous rotary vacuum filter press
    d. None of the above

13. **Select a genuine criteria for the selection of a filter press?**
    a. Equipment life   b. Availability of floor area
    c. Chemical reactivity   d. All of above

14. **Rate of filtration depends upon?**
    a. Compressibility factor of the filtrate
    b. Pressure drop
    c. Both a and b
    d. None

15. **What is adding of cellulose in the pulping of certain fruit juices called? Was its addition in the process of filtration is right?**
    a. Filter cloth, yes   b. Filter aid, yes
    c. Filter cloth, no   d. Filter aid, no

16. **Continuous rotary vacuum filter press has a:**
    Statement 1: High labour cost.
    Statement 2: High clogging.
    a. True, False   b. True, True
    c. False, False   d. False, True

Centrifugation

Nikita and Yasmin Sultana

Centrifugation is defined as a process used for separating the constituents present in dispersion with the help of centrifugal force. Centrifugal force is applied to provide the driving force for two operations, i.e. to create a pressure difference in the filtration process and to replace gravitational force in the sedimentation process. Centrifugation provides a convenient method for the separation of either two immiscible liquids or a solid from the liquid.

Centrifugation is based on the well-known principle that an object that is rotated about a centre point at a constant radial distance from that point is acted upon by a centrifugal force.

OBJECTIVES

- To evaluate the biopharmaceutical drug dosage forms
- To separate the desired component from the sample product
- To assess the emulsions and suspensions
- To produce biological products.

APPLICATIONS

Biopharmaceutical evaluation of drugs: Centrifugation method is used for the separation of the drugs as the drugs are usually present in the form of colloidal dispersions in the biological fluids like blood, tissue fluids and urine and thus, it is used for the pharmacokinetic and bioequivalence estimation of drug.

Production of bulk drugs: Centrifugation is useful for separating the crystalline drugs like aspirin from the mother liquor as the traces of the mother liquor are removed, resulting in the free flowing sample with no effervescence.

Determination of molecular weight of colloids: Molecular weight of the polymers cannot be ascertained by normal methods and therefore, ultra-centrifugation methods are used for the evaluation of molecular weight of serum albumin, methylcellulose, and insulin. Also, ultracentrifugation methods are used for establishing the degree of homogeneity of the sample. For example, insulin is comprised of two polypeptide chains and is a monodisperse protein whereas gelatin is found to have fragments of molecular weight 10,000 to 1,00,000 and is polydisperse protein.

Assessment of emulsions and suspension: It is considered to be the instant verifiable test parameter for the estimation of emulsions and suspensions. Usually, creaming is a gradual process in case of emulsions and it can be accelerated by generating stress condition with the help of centrifuge. A stable emulsion should not separate even after, if is centrifuged at 2000–3000 rpm at room temperature.

Production of biological products: Most of the proteinaceous drugs are present as colloidal dispersions in water and thus, it is difficult to produce them at a large scale using common methods. Therefore, the isolation of these components is carried out by applying centrifugal force. Insulin in the pure form can be isolated by selective precipitation of other proteins and consequently their separation by ultracentrifugation. Blood cells are also separated from blood using centrifugation method.

PRINCIPLES AND THEORY OF CENTRIFUGATION

Particles having the size above 5 µm sediment at the bottom due to gravity. In such a case, separation of solids is possible by simple filtration. If particles are of the order of 5 µm or less they undergo Brownian motion and hence, they do not sediment under gravity. Therefore, it requires a strong centrifugal force to separate them. The sedimentation also depends on the densities of the dispersed phase and dispersion medium. If the difference in the densities of these phases is less, separation will be very difficult. By applying centrifugal force, it is possible to facilitate the separation process. The operations using centrifugal force are described by equation including the gravitational constant. It is convenient to measure the centrifugal force in terms of a ratio to the gravitational force and it is known as the centrifugal effect. The centrifugal effect is obtained as follows: suppose a body of mass m, rotating in a circular path of radius r, at a velocity v (Fig. 10.1) and the force acting on the body in a radial direction is given as:

$$F = \frac{mv^2}{r}$$

where,
   F = Centrifugal force
   m = Mass of body
   v = Velocity of body
   r = Radius of circle of rotation

The same body when acted upon by gravitational force:

$$G = mg$$

where,
   G = Gravitational force
   g = Gravitational constant

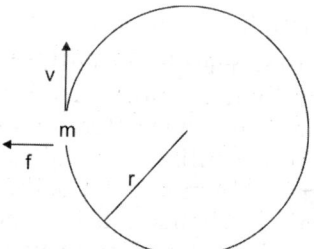

Fig. 10.1: Principles of centrifugation

The centrifugal effect is ratio of the two forces, so that:

$$C = \frac{F}{G}$$

$$= \frac{mv^2}{mgr}$$

$$= \frac{v^2}{gr}$$

$$v = 2\pi rn$$

where,

n = Speed of rotation

$\therefore$

$$\frac{F}{G} = \frac{(2\pi rn)^2}{gr}$$

$$= \frac{4\pi^2 r^2 n^2}{gr}$$

$$= \frac{2(2r)\pi^2 n^2 r}{gr}$$

$$C = \frac{2\pi^2 n^2 d}{g}$$

where,

d = Diameter of rotation

The gravitational constant has a value of 9.807 m/s^2, so the above equation may be simplified as, provided that n is expressed in second^{-1} and d in meter.

$$\text{Centrifugal effect} = 2.013\ n^2 d$$

From the above equations, the important conclusion can be drawn that the centrifugal effect is directly proportional to the diameter and is also proportional to the square of the speed of rotation. Thus, when it is necessary to increase the centrifugal effect, it is of great advantage to use a centrifuge of the same size at a higher speed, rather than use a large centrifuge at the same speed of rotation.

Centrifuges can be classified based on their mechanisms of separation:

Sedimentation centrifuge

It is a centrifuge that produces sedimentation of solids which are based on the difference in the densities of two or more phases of the mixture. The efficiency depends on the velocity of rotation to which the mixture is subjected.

Filtration centrifuge

In this centrifuge solid pass through the porous medium, i.e. based on the difference in the densities of the solid and liquid phases. In it, the container contains a porous wall through which the liquid phase may pass and on which the solid phase is retained.

INDUSTRIAL CENTRIFUGES

PERFORATED BASKET CENTRIFUGE

Principle: It is a filtration centrifuge. The separation occurs through a perforated wall which is based on the difference in the densities of solid and liquid phases. The bowl consists of a perforated side wall. During centrifugation, the liquid phase passes through the perforated wall, whereas solid phase is retained in the bowl and the solid is removed after cutting the sediment by blade after stopping the centrifuge.

Construction: It can either be under-driven or over-driven. In the under-driven perforated basket centrifuge, the basket is mounted above driving shaft, conversely, if the basket is suspended from a shaft, it is described as over-driven. This under-driven perforated basket centrifuge consists of a basket that is made of steel sometimes covered with vulcanite/lead/copper or any other suitable metal. The basket material of construction should be such that it offers the greatest resistance to corrosion. The basket may have a diameter of 0.90 meters and a capacity of 0.085 metre cube. The diameter of the perforations should be selected on the basis of size of crystals to be separated. In case, the size of perforations is bigger than that of particles, a filter cloth is employed (Fig. 10.2).

The basket is suspended on vertical shaft and is driven by a motor using suitable power systems, such as belt pulleys, water turbines and electric motors. The basket may require about 5 kilowatt power for starting and 2 kilowatt for running. Sometimes, steel hoops are used externally to strengthen the basket. Surrounding the basket, a stationary casing is provided which collects the filtrate and discharges it at the outlet.

Working: The material is kept in a stationary basket. The amount of material should be optimum in order to avoid the strain on the basket and loading is done in such a way such that it is evenly distributed. Power is applied to rotate the basket and maximum speed must be attained quickly. The basket runs at 1000 rpm. During centrifugation process the liquid passes through the perforated wall, while the solid retains in the basket only. The liquid leaves the basket and is collected at the outlet. The cake is then spun to dry and sometimes high speeds are used to dry the cake completely. After a definite period of time power is turned off and centrifuge is

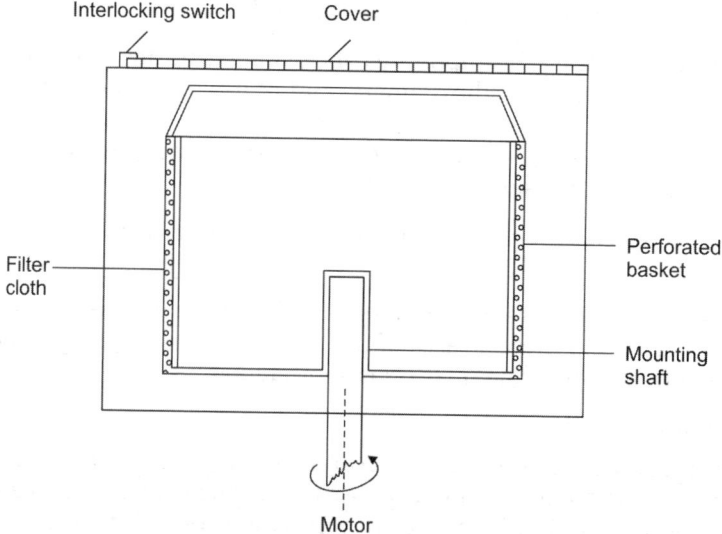

Fig. 10.2: Construction of perforated basket centrifuge

stopped by applying brakes. The basket is brought to rest and the solid cake is cut with the blade and unloaded manually.

Uses

- It is used to separate crystalline drugs from mother liquor as the free flowing product is obtained because mother liquor can be removed completely
- It is used to separate unwanted solids from a liquid
- It is used for the separation of the sugar crystals.

Advantages

- It is very compact and occupies very little floor space
- It can handle slurries with high proportion of solids
- The final product has very low moisture content and in this method, the dissolved solids are separated from the cake
- It is a rapid process.

Disadvantages

- The entire process is complicated leading to high labour costs
- It is a batch process
- Prolonged operation may lead to considerable wear and tear of the equipment and also the solids may form hard cake due to centrifugal force which is difficult to remove simultaneously.

NON-PERFORATED BASKET CENTRIFUGE

Principle: It is a kind of sedimentation centrifuge. It is based on the difference in the densities of liquid and solid phases without a porous barrier. The bowl consists of a non-perforated side wall. During the centrifugation process liquid remains at the top and is removed with the help of skimming tube while solid phase is retained on the sides of the basket.

   Construction: It consists of a basket which is made of steel or any other suitable metal. The basket is kept suspended on a vertical shaft which is driven by a motor using power system (Fig. 10.3).

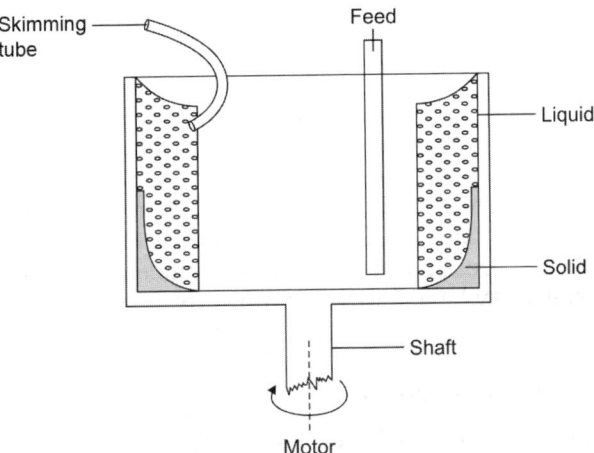

Fig. 10.3: Construction of non-perforated basket centrifuge

Working: During the centrifugation process, the suspension is fed continuously into the basket and liquid remains at the top while solid phase is retained on the sides of the basket. The liquid is removed with the help of a skimming tube. The operation is stopped when the suitable depth of solids is deposited on the walls of the basket and is scrapped off by hand or using a scrapper blade.

Uses

It is useful when the deposited solids offer high resistance to the flow of liquid.

Advantages

- It enables the separation of solids and liquids of different densities
- The separation is more effective as there is no porous barrier due to the non-perforated basket.

Disadvantage

It is a batch process.

SEMI-CONTINUOUS CENTRIFUGE OR SHORT CYCLE AUTOMATIC BATCH CENTRIFUGE

Principle: It is a filtration centrifuge. The separation is achieved through a perforated wall-based on the difference in the densities of liquid and solid phases. The bowl contains a perforated side-wall. During the centrifugation process, the liquid phase passes through the perforated wall whereas the solid phase is retained in the bowl. The solid is then washed and removed by cutting the sediment using a blade.

Construction: It consists of vertical perforated basket supported from a horizontal shaft driven by a motor. From the open side of the basket the horizontal pipes for the feed and washing pipe are made at the centre of the basket. A feeler rides over the feed which is connected to the diaphragm valve through air supply. The feeler controls the thickness of the feed. Hydraulic cylinder attachment is made in such a way that the discharge chute enters from the sides of the basket, when discharge of crystals is desirable (Fig. 10.4).

Working: During centrifugation, the slurry is introduced from the side pipe and passes through the perforated wall and the perforated basket is allowed to rotate. The solids remain in the basket while filtrate leaves the basket, which is collected at outlet and the cake is washed with water. The wash is removed from the basket through the filtrate outlet.

When the desired thickness is achieved then, the feeler cuts off the air supply to a diaphragm valve that helps in automatically shuts off the entry of slurry. The hydraulic cylinder is actuated that lifts the knife along with the discharge. The knife does not cut the cake completely down to the screen but leaves a layer of crystals that acts as a filter medium for further separation in the next cycle. The air supply mechanisms, diaphragm valve controls all stops through a timer therefore, the entire cycle is semi-automatic. The discharge crystals may have 2 to 4% of moisture.

Uses

- It is used for separation of colloids
- It is used for purification of insulin by selective precipitation
- It is used for determining efficacy of blood samples.

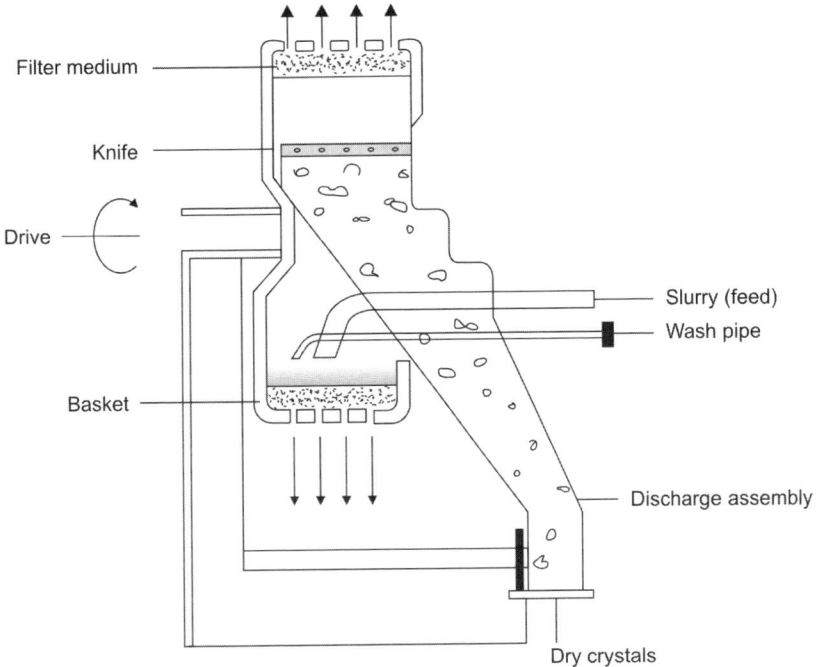

Fig. 10.4: Construction of semi-continuous centrifuge

Advantages
- It can be used when the solids can be drained fast from the bowl
- It is fast and effective.

Disadvantages
- Considerable breakage of crystals is possible during discharge
- The construction of centrifuge involves moving parts and its functioning is complicated.

SUPER CENTRIFUGE

Super centrifuge is a continuous centrifuge used for separating two immiscible liquid phases.

Principle: It is a sedimentation centrifuge in which the separation is based on the difference in the densities between two immiscible liquids. Centrifugation is done in the bowl of small centrifuge. During the process, the heavier liquid is thrown against the wall, whereas the lighter liquid remains as an inner layer. The two layers are simultaneously separated using modified weirs (Fig. 10.5).

Construction: It contains a long hollow cylindrical bowl of small diameter and is suspended from a flexible spindle at the top. It is guided at the bottom with the help of loose-fit bushing that can be rotated on its longitudinal axis. At the bottom, a provision is made for the feed inlet by a pressure system. At different heights, two liquid outlets are provided on the top of the bowl and are attached by modified weirs.

Working: The centrifuge is allowed to rotate at high speed usually at speed of 2000 revolutions per minute with the help of drive assembly. The feed is introduced through

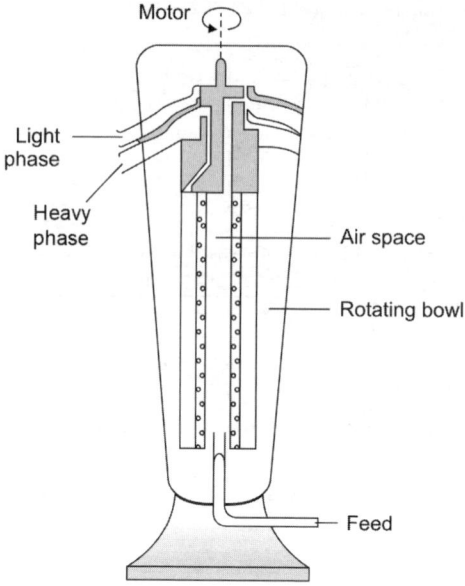

Fig. 10.5: Construction of super centrifuge

the feed inlet at the bottom using a pressure system. During the centrifugation process the two liquid phases separate on the basis of difference in the densities of the liquids. The heavier liquid is thrown against the wall whereas the lighter liquid remains and form an inner layer. Both the liquids rise to the top of the vertical bowl.

The liquid-liquid interface is maintained by a hydraulic balance. These two layers are simultaneously removed as two liquids, i.e. light phase and heavy phase, separately from different heights through modified weirs. Thus, the super centrifuge can work for continuous separation of immiscible liquid phases.

Use
- It is used for separating liquid phases of emulsions in foods and pharmaceuticals
- It is used for purification of diesel process fuel oil
- It is used in various industrial applications, such as soda solution, gum clarification, etc.
- Removal of oversize pigments from paints
- Fraction of blood human plasma
- Harvesting biomass.

Advantages
- Continuous process
- Can be used to separate two immiscible liquids
- It is a rapid process.

Disadvantages
- It is costly
- Has high energy consumption
- It is difficult to clean and maintain.

VERY SHORT QUESTIONS

1. Write the principle of sedimentation and centrifugation.

2. How frictional force influences centrifugation process?

3. How to safeguard centrifuge?

4. Write the applications of centrifugation.

5. Define following terms: Centrifugation, sedimentation velocity, RFC, RPM.

SHORT QUESTIONS

1. What is centrifugation? Enlist its objectives.

2. Derive the equation to establish relationship between RCF and RPM.

3. Explain the principle of super centrifuge and enlist its applications.

4. Differentiate between perforated and non-perforated centrifuge with the help of suitable diagram.

5. What is meant by under driven filtration type centrifuge?

LONG QUESTIONS

1. Explain the principle and theory of centrifugation.

2. Explain the principle, construction, working, uses, advantages and disadvantages of centrifuge used for size separation of slurry containing high percentage of solids.

3. Explain the principle, construction, working, uses, advantages and disadvantages of centrifuge used for size separation of emulsion.

4. Write a detailed note on semi continuous centrifuge.

MULTIPLE CHOICE QUESTIONS

1. **Cell fractionation is having a primary objective:**
   a. To crack the cell wall so that the cytoplasmic contents can be released
   b. To identify the enzymes outside the organelles
   c. To view the structure of cell membranes
   d. To separate the major organelles so that their particular functions can be determined

2. **........................... is widely used to separate and purify biological particles in a liquid medium under applied centrifugal force.**
   a. Centrifugation
   b. Microscope
   c. pH meter
   d. None of the above

3. .... type of rotors, the sample tubes are loaded into individual buckets that hang vertically while the rotor is at rest. When the rotor begins to rotate the buckets swing out to a horizontal position?
   a. Swinging-bucket
   b. Fixed-angle
   c. Vertical
   d. None of the above

4. The type of centrifuge that is under driven
   a. Horizontal continuous centrifuge
   b. Perforated basket centrifuge
   c. Semi continous centrifuge
   d. None of the above

5. .... factors does not affect separation process.
   a. Time
   b. Nature of slurry
   c. Speed
   d. Temperature

6. Factors important while designing a centrifugation protocol are:
   a. The more massive a biological particle is, the faster it moves in a centrifugal field
   b. The denser the biological buffer system is, the slower the particle will move in a centrifugal field
   c. The greater the frictional coefficient is, the slower a particle will move
   d. All of the above

7. RPM stands for:
   a. Round per minutes
   b. Right per minutes
   c. Revolution per minutes
   d. Rotation per minutes

8. In equation, $G = \omega^2 r$ where ω equals to:
   a. Radial distance from the axis of rotation
   b. Centrifugal force
   c. Angular velocity
   d. None of the above

9. Separation of analyte depends on:
   a. Size
   b. Shape
   c. Density
   d. All of the above

10. The technique used to separate molecule with same size of particles (M) but different shapes are:
    a. Zones of equal density centrifugation
    b. Preparative ultracentrifuges
    c. None of the above
    d. All of the above

11. For a sedimentation type .... is a condition.
    a. Basket is non-perforated
    b. Basket is perforated
    c. Containing filter aid
    d. Containing filter medium

12. Centrifuges are used for the analysis of dosage forms in terms of stability:
    a. Chemical stability
    b. Physical stability
    c. Thermal stability
    d. Photostability

Pharmaceutical Plant Construction

Syed Mahmood, Shakeeb Ahmed and Yasmin Sultana

FACTORS AFFECTING SELECTION OF MATERIALS FOR PHARMACEUTICAL PLANT

The chemical, physical, mechanical and economical factors have to be considered while selecting various materials for pharmaceutical plant construction. As this factor place an important role in the construction as well as in the production also. "As these factors play an important role in the construction as well as production."

Chemical Properties

There should be no chemical reaction between materials being processed and part of the machine. Two aspects of chemical action must be considered under this section, namely:

1. The contamination of the product by the material of the plant
2. The effect on the material of the plant by the drugs and chemical processed.

Impurities have considerable physiological effects and even in traces, cause the product to decompose. For example, presence of heavy metals inactivate the penicillin. The appearance might also be affected due to changes in colour due to contamination. The contamination from some materials may be innocuous, the products being non-toxic.

With increasing knowledge new materials are being employed which are resistant to the attacked by acids, alkalis, oxidising agents, tannins, etc. and new alloys having different physical and chemical properties are developed to meet the problems of chemical reactions.

Physical Properties

Hardness, density, melting range, thermal expansion coefficient, thermal conductivity, electrical resistivity and tensile modulus of elasticity are some of the typical physical constant considered to assess the resistibility of the metals or an alloy in the pharmaceutical plant construction. With the help of the above-mentioned physical constant, the following physical properties are studied for a metal, non-metal and alloy.

Mechanical Strength

In an operation, when the flowing liquid or gas contains solid particles that are harder than the metal surface of the machine, erosion will occur. Thus harder materials help to prevent erosion attack.

Weight

The lightness of a machine or its components, without significant compromise on efficiency, is preferable. A heavy machine poses problems in transferring from one place to other. A machine may have to be shifted from one place to other to utilise its services for a number of operations in different sections located close by or for repairing purpose.

Ease of Fabrication

The material selected for constructing a plant must be easily fabricated to the desired shape. If a metal is brittle, it tends to break easily and is difficult to machine. For example, stainless steel can be more easily fabricated into the machine than cast iron.

Expansivity

This is of great importance among physical properties. A surprisingly large numbers of metal failure at elevated temperature are the result of excessive thermal stress originating from a constituent of the metal during heating or cooling. Such an expansion in the case of hindered contraction can cause rupturing.

Thermal Expansion

The design of plants becomes greatly complicated if the material has a high coefficient of expansion which leads to increase stresses and the risk of fracture also as the temperature changes. The material is required to maintain size and shape of equipment at a working temperature.

Thermal Conductivity

In plants, such as stills and evaporators, dryer, heat exchanger, a good thermal conductivity is desirable. The resistant film highly retards the heat transfer process, e.g. iron, glass or graphite is used in the fabrication of heat exchangers, to affect the heat transfer.

Wear and Tear

When there is the possibility of friction between the moving parts of the equipment, this property becomes important. It may cause the contamination of the processed material. The risk of contamination is highly found due to wear of ceramic/iron equipment.

Ease of Cleaning

A machine might have to be cleaned between or after the operation. The surface must be smooth for efficient and easy cleaning.

Transparency

A certain part of a machine might be essentially transparent to view any operation going on inside. The transparent material employed, e.g. glass or any synthetic material must be able to resist the strains of the operation.

Mechanical Properties

Typical mechanical properties studied include yield strength, tensile strength and elongation of a metal or its alloy. For non-metals, a few additional mechanical properties include compression strength, impact strength, etc.

Based on the above measurements the mechanical properties considered in the selection of a metal, non-metal and alloy include creep, rupture and short-time strength, various forms of ductility as well as resistance to impact and fatigue stresses. Creep strength and stress rupture are usually of great interest to designers of stationary equipment, such as vessels and furnaces. Stress rupture is another important consideration at high temperature since, it relates to stress and time to produce rupture.

Economics in Material Selection

Purchasing and maintenance cost of the plant must be economical. The main concern is not simply to obtain a cheap material. Better quality product or plant material will be more economical. Any cost estimation should include the following:

1. Total material cost
2. Labour cost in installation
3. Maintenance cost
4. Replacement costs.

CLASSIFICATION OF MATERIALS OF PLANT CONSTRUCTION

Materials of plant construction can be classified as follows:

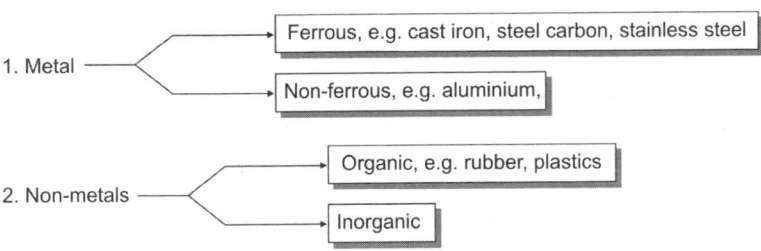

Metals

Ferrous Metals

Cast iron: It consists of iron with a proportion of carbon. The amount of carbon varies, giving products with different properties. Its characteristics may also be changed by alloying with other elements, e.g. silicon, nickel, chromium. Silicon alloys have found more resistant to acids (e.g. concentrated sulphuric acid, nitric acid) and dilute alkalis. They are very hard and brittle so they cannot be machined.

It is attacked by dilute sulphuric acid and nitric acid and by both dilute and concentrated hydrochloric acid. At high temperature, it is attacked by ammonium salts. It also acts with tannins. It is very cheap metal. It is commonly used as the supports for plants, for the jackets of the steam pan, etc. It is also used as a coating material.

Steels: Mild steel contains only a small percentage of carbon. It has greater mechanical strength and is less brittle. Their resistance property against attack by chemicals is similar to that of cast iron. Mild steel is used in the chemical and pharmaceutical industries. It is found to be used for supporting structures, such as girders and bases for plant vessels, vessels, pipelines and smaller accessories—nuts and bolts.

Stainless steel: These are steel alloys mostly with nickel and chromium. They are highly resistant to corrosion. Stainless steel containing 18 percentage of chromium and 8 percentage of nickel is known as "18/8 stainless steel" is used in pharmaceutical industries. Plants of various shape and size can be made from stainless steel. The problem of corrosion can be prevented by reducing the carbon content or the inclusion of stabilisers, such as titanium, molybdenum or niobium. Stainless steel can be used for most pharmaceutical plant, including storage and extraction vessels, evaporators and fermentation vessels. Small apparatus commonly made from stainless steel includes funnels, buckets, measuring vessels and shovels. Sink and bench tops are also made of stainless steels. It is a costly metal, so often it is excluded from the use.

Non-ferrous Metals

Copper: It is a malleable and ductile metal, so can be easily fabricated. Its thermal conductivity is 8 times greater than stainless steel, but it is corroded by oxidising agents. It is also attacked by all concentration of nitric acid, hot concentrated sulphuric acid and hydrochloric acid and by some organic acids. Ammonia reacts with it readily to form blue cupro-ammonium compounds. Many drug constituents react with it, so, for this reason, copper is usually protected by a lining of tin when used for pharmaceutical plants. It is used for evaporators, pans of various kinds, stills, fractionating columns and so on. Copper piping is easy to make so it is extensively used for services, such as cold water, gas, vacuum and low-pressure steam.

Aluminium: Aluminium has good corrosion resistance property. It is resistant to oxidising conditions because it forms a compact oxide film. It is also resistant to strong nitric acid, caustic alkalis, mercury and its salts, but is attacked by mineral acids. Pure aluminium is soft in nature but more corrosion resistant than most of its alloy such as Duralumin. Alloys of aluminium can be formed with a small percentage of manganese, magnesium or silicon. Aluminium plants are easily fabricated and have excellent thermal conductivity. It is a non-toxic metal. It is used to construct the plants that are used in the production of medicines, culture media and antibiotics. It shows very low density due to which it is mostly useful for the preparation of transport containers, such as drums, barrels, roads and rail tankers.

Lead: It is corrosion resistant material and can be easily converted into a complicated shape. It has little use in pharmaceutical industries due to the risk of contamination by presence of poisonous lead salts, but used for cold water pipes, waste pipe and also in dilution tanks for laboratories.

Tin: Tin is a highly resistant material to a great variety of substances. Its salts are non-toxic in nature, so it is widely used throughout the food industry. It is mainly used to provide a protective coating for steel, copper, brass, etc.

Silver: It is a very expensive metal. It is mainly used to coat the materials. It is found to be resistant to organic acids and their salts and has highly malleable and ductile properties. It also shows higher thermal conductivity than other metals.

Nickel: It is resistant to oxidation and alkali but can be attacked by concentrated acids and dilute minerals. It shows resistant to phenols and weak organic acids, such as citric acid, tartaric acid and stearic acid. Its salts are non-toxic and are useful for plants in pans, tanks, mixers, valves, and pumps. Monel metal is harder and resistant than nickel and can be replaced by steel where corrosion resistance is required.

Chromium: It is very hard, resistant to corrosion and this is the reason it is not normally used as a material of plant construction. It forms a resistant alloy with nickel. It is mostly used in the manufacturing of stainless steel and also used for plating to protect the steel.

Non-metals

Glass: Glass is very resistant to corrosion and is widely used for small-scale apparatus. The ordinary soda-lime glass is used for bottles and other cheap articles but is not satisfactory for large scale plants or for containers where alkali contamination might be a serious drawback. For these purpose borosilicate glass is used. Borosilicate glass is less brittle, has a low thermal expansion and can be used with a safety over wide temperature ranges. However, its thermal conductivity is low therefore it should be heated gradually to avoid fracture. A special advantage of glass is that it can be easily cleaned, sterilised and also, the content of vessels can be readily examined for colour and clarity. Glass pipeline is useful for transporting liquids from one stage to other. All-glass stills are used for preparing water for injection and other distilled preparations. Glass fibres are excellent for heat insulation or refrigeration plant. Such fibre is used for filtering air asepsis room. Woven fibre may be used for filter cloths.

Stone ware: Ceramics are reasonably cheap, but weight, low thermal conductivity, and fragility give only a low resistance to mechanical and thermal shock. Corrosion resistance is usually due to a surface glaze which may become chipped. Ceramics are used in small scale to produce pipeline, tanks, vessels and filters.

Asbestos: It is a poor conductor of heat. It may be used for heat insulation. Since, it is extremely inert, it can be used for pipelining and for pipe joining. It is fibrous material and may be woven into cloth for filters.

Organic

- *Rubber*: It may be used for lining and coating. It swells in contact with oils. It is subject to oxidation and is attacked by some organic solvents. The synthetic rubber that has greater resistance has been developed.
- *Plastics*: It is a phenolic resin with various inert fillers selected for their particular purpose. It may be machined, welded and worked in other ways and is resistant to corrosion. Its weight is about is one-quarter that of iron. It may be attacked by oxidising substances and strong alkalis. Any item may be constructed from this material like vessels, pipes, fittings, valves, pumps, fans, ducts, filter presses.

Polyethene and polypropylene chloride (PVC) are similar material and are rigid or flexible depending upon the amount of rubber added. Metallic surface may be protected from corrosion by coating them with plastics of the polyethene or polypropylene chloride. Special transparent plastic also used to guards for moving parts of machinery and asepsis screen. Nylon and polypropylene chloride fibre may be woven into filter cloth.

CORROSION

Corrosion is defined as a destructive attack or gradual destruction of the materials like metals, semiconductor, insulators and polymers by chemical or electrochemical reaction with the environment. It means that breaking down of essential properties in a material due to chemical reactions with its surroundings, therefore a loss of electrons of metals reacting with water and oxygen. It is also defined as irreversible change or damage of materials due to chemical and electrochemical reaction. Figure 11.1 showing a diagram of typical corrosion.

The environment can be a gas phase with or without moisture and aqueous or non-aqueous electrolyte. Pharmaceutical plant materials are very liable for the corrosion as the majority of the equipment's and plant construction depends on the metals. The corrosion (chemical and electrochemical reaction) processes which occur at the surface and may involve the bulk of the materials and the liquid phase or gas contacting gas.

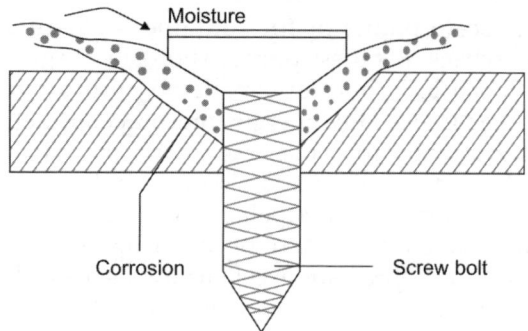

Fig. 11.1: Corrosion

Physical causes which are responsible for the deterioration of the materials are termed galling, wearing or erosion. Non-metals are not counted in process of the corrosion. Wood may split or decay, plastic may swell or crack, cement may leach away and granite may erode but term corrosion is restricted to chemical attack of the metals. Ferrous compounds have being termed with the special terminology called rusting, it applies to the corrosion of iron or iron-base alloys with the formation of corrosion products consisting largely of hydrous ferric oxides. Rusting as it produces iron oxide; it is a good example of electrochemical corrosion. Corrosion is a process by chemical change brings a change in the metal, so in order to understand it, the basic principle of the chemistry of chemical and physical metallurgy of metals must be known (Fig. 11.2).

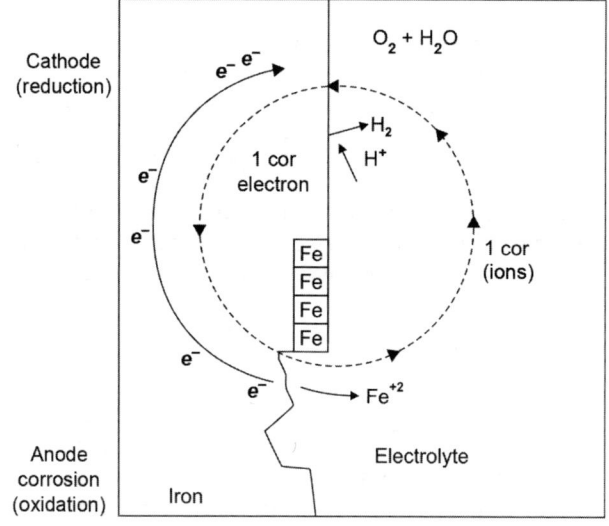

Fig. 11.2: Anodic and cathodic reaction

TYPES OF CORROSION

The chemical and electrochemical process that result in deterioration in form of corrosion of the materials decide is different types which can be classified as:

   I. **General attack corrosion:** It is also known as uniform attack corrosion and is most common type of corrosion and is caused by electrochemical or chemical reaction, it proceeds more or less uniformly over an exposed surface without appreciable localisation, and it turns out in the deterioration of entire exposed surface. It leads to relatively uniform thinning on sheet and plate materials and general thinning on one side or the other (or both) for pipe and tubing, characterised by rusting and peeling effect of the metals thin films and keep on depleting the metal take place until failure. Other examples of this type of corrosion are discolouration of the metal surface which also includes polished surface or their dulling. Cleaning or etching by acid can also leads to corrosion. It is recognised by a roughening of the surface and usually by the presence of corrosion products. This type of corrosion brings for the greatest amount of metal destruction by corrosion but is predictable, manageable and often preventable considered as a safe form of corrosion. To control this type of corrosions usually cathodic protection, use of coating or oil paints is used. The metal coatings which are used in protection are copper and titanium which are rusting free metals known. In some cases, depending upon the metals to be protected gold and silver coating is applied.

II. **Localised corrosion:** It happens at the specific targets area of the metal or polymer structure. This type of corrosion is metal depended on corrosion with respect to the environmental factor, it is an intense attack at localizes sites on the surface of a component, while the remaining area of the surface of the corroded material decays slowly. This happens due to the inherent property of the components materials and its chemical reaction with environment like in the creation of protective film oxide. Usually, this corrosion takes place at a site where the corrosion protective coating ends and reduces. Other types of localising corrosion known:

   a. **Crevice corrosion:** It takes place at a shielded area or under the surface or at the joint assembly and at crevice. For example, acidic conditions or a depletion of oxygen in a metal hole or cracks may lead to crevice corrosion.

   b. **Pitting corrosion:** It takes place at the free and open surface of the materials which become liable to the corrosion after coming in contact with certain chemicals. This corrosion result in metals holes surface, these holes are also described as cavities with a surface diameter as same the depth. This corrosion happens in a small area so in this case, they are less detected.

   c. **Intergranular corrosion:** It is a limited corrosion which is not so dangerous for the metal, but in some grains, boundaries are reactive compared to the matrix and can result in corrosion.

III. **Galvanic corrosion:** This corrosion takes place when one metal which is liable for corrosion comes in touch with another metal and they are in electrical contact in the presence of a corrosive electrolyte. Every metal has different electro-potential, so in this, an anode and cathode form when the electrolyte is present. The driving force from dissimilar metals is in term of electropotential cause and accelerate attack on the anode membrane of galvanic couple. The anode metal when comes in contact with the electrolyte (which provides a passage for ion migration) dissolves and deposits on the cathodic metals, to form a protective layer against corrosion. An example of galvanic corrosion is the technique of cleaning silverware by immersion of the silver and a piece of aluminium in an electrolytic bath (usually sodium bicarbonate) is an example of galvanic corrosion.

Three common factor needed are:

a. Electrochemically dissimilar metals must be present

b. The metals should expose to an electrolyte

c. There must be electrically in contact with each other.

IV. **Flow-assisted corrosion (FAC):** As by its name flow-assisted/accelerated, when the protective layer of poorly soluble oxide on the surface of the material is dissolved or damaged by external environmental factors, such as water and the wind, the resultant will be the corrosion of the underlying material. This type of corrosion affects carbon steel piping carrying ultra-pure, deoxygenated water or wet steam. It also results in the formation of other derived corrosion like impingement, cavitation and erosion-assisted corrosion.

V. **Environmental cracking:** This type of corrosion results mainly from the environmental related factors that can affect the metal. There are many types of environmental cracking that take place by chemical, temperature and stress-related conditions. They are hydrogen induced cracking, stress corrosion cracking (SCC), liquid metal embrittlement and corrosion fatigue.

VI. **De-Alloying:** It is also called selective corrosion or selective leaching. The demetallization process happens at the solid solution alloys when they are exposed to the particular conditions a component of the alloys is leached out from the materials of a particular element, making that area susceptible to further corrosion. The high distance between the galvanic series of the alloy and its metals makes that material more susceptible for the demetallization. The most common elements undergo selective leaching are aluminium, iron, zinc, cobalt, chromium, etc. A suitable and most common example of de-alloying is dezincification. In this selective leaching of zinc from unstabilize brass alloys containing more than 15–20% zinc when exposed to moisture and oxygen, which result in the formation of porous copper structure. In this zinc is dissolves with brass in the leftover solution and copper add as a new plate from the solution (replating). This process can also cause by water containing sulphur, CO_2, and O_2. In order to protect the demetallization of zinc, arsenic or tin can be added to the brass at the time formation of the alloy or electroplating done with gunmetal. The dezincification-resistant brass (DZR) or brass C352 is an alloy used to make pipe fitting for potable water transportation. Graphitic-iron leaching is another example of this type of corrosion where iron from grey cast iron, in this iron leach out and graphite grains, remains intact. It can be reduced by using alloying the casting iron with nickel.

VII. **Fretting corrosion:** This type corrosion results from the repeated wearing and related processes which result in asperities (uneven, roughness and ruggedness) of the contact surface. They form pits and small holes on the surface of the machines especially which have rotation and impact machinery, bolted assemblies and bearing, e.g. Ball mill, V-cone blender, orbital shaker, planetary shaker, the mixture used in the larger scale of mixing of powder. This type of corrosion attacks the surface layer quality by producing an increased susceptibility to the surface roughness and micro-pits, which decreases the fatigue strength of the machinery.

VIII. **High-temperature corrosion:** As the name suggests the high-temperature corrosion is the cause of high temperature produced by hot gases and when they come in contact with certain contaminants. Machineries that are affected by this type of corrosion are turbines, petrochemical related engines, furnaces, etc. Fuels used in industries contain vanadium or sulphates, and during burning those at very high-temperature combustion form some compounds with low melting points. These low melting points compound is very corrosive towards metal alloys, stainless steel and high temperatures. The high-temperature corrosion can also happen by oxidation, carbonisation and sulfidation.

FACTORS INFLUENCING CORROSION PROCESS

Corrosion can be increased and influenced by many factors, including its rate and spreadability with time. For a corrosion to occur and to complete a corrosion cell a cathode (–), an anode (+), an electrolyte and a metallic conductor are required. Corrosion rate is divided into two parts, factors responsible for corrosive environment and affecting the metal and subdivided into other important factors that influence corrosion rates are:

- *Temperature*: With increase in temperature the corrosion rate increase, hot and warmer temperature increase corrosion rate as compared to the colder temperature.

- *Chemical salt*: The potential power of electrolyte can change the rate of corrosion drastically. When chemical shift increases, it also increases efficiency (conductance) of the electrolyte with reference to anode and cathode. The common examples in pharmaceutical industries of chemical shifting and resultant corrosion is when some machinery requires the chemical treatment with a hygroscopic compound like magnesium chloride, sodium chloride, calcium chloride, etc. They retain moisture from the environment, so they expose the material to the corrosion and also increases the rate of corrosion.

- *Oxygen*: Oxygen is also responsible for increasing the rate of corrosion as observed in the case of water (moisture). In absence of oxygen, corrosion can also takes place but the degree of intensity is slow as compared to the presence of oxygen.

- *Humidity*: Humidity is moisture that results in a rate of corrosion, usually the rate of increase is observed. Atmospheric exposure is the time of wetting that a metal undergoes and initiate or continue the process of corrosion.

- *Pollutants*: That results from the environmental factor and can lead to corrosion like dust, acid rain, chlorides and other corrosive chemicals can initiate the corrosion.

CORROSION CAUSES AND ITS MECHANISM

The causes of corrosion can be understood by the mainly two parameters that are Gibbs free energy and Pilling-Bedworth ratio.

Gibbs's Free Energy (ΔG)

Changes in Gibbs energy (G), will initiate the reaction. As the reaction will proceed, the direction will follow where, the G is low. As Gibb's free energy shifts to more negative the greater the intensity of the reaction to proceed. Gibb's free energy can be defined as a thermodynamic potential that measures the maximum or reversible work that may be performed by a thermodynamic system at a constant pressure and temperature or which can be also said as isobaric and isothermal respectively. It is a maximum amount of non-expansion work that can be extracted from a thermodynamically closed system in which they exchange heat and work with its surrounding environment, but not matter. The process of changing the system from initial stability to final stability, the change in free Gibbs energy ΔG is always the work exchanged by the system with its surroundings, minus the work of pressure forces, the process happens as the reversible transformation of the system from the initial state to the final state. American mathematician Josiah Willard Gibbs, discovered this phenomenon in 1873, Gibbs described this "available energy" as "the greatest amount of mechanical work which can be obtained from a given quantity of a certain substance in a given initial state, without increasing its total volume or allowing heat to pass to or from external bodies, except such as at the close of the processes are left in their initial condition". The SI unit of Gibb's free energy is kJ/mol.

Some reactions related to Gibb's free energy and how the reaction of corrosion proceeds, consider the following reaction at 25°C.

$$Mg + H_2O \text{ (1)} + \tfrac{1}{2}O_2 \text{ (g)} \rightarrow Mg(OH)_2 \text{ (S)} \qquad \Delta G° = -596,600 \text{ J}$$

Greater negative value of $\Delta G°$, result in more reaction of magnesium to react with oxygen and water.

$$Cu + H_2O \text{ (1)} + \tfrac{1}{2}O_2 \text{ (g)} \rightarrow Cu(OH)_2 \text{ (S)} \qquad \Delta G° = -119,700 \text{ J}$$

The reaction intensity of this reaction is less, hence the copper (Cu) corrosion reaction is slow.

In another case,

$$Au + \tfrac{3}{2}H_2O \text{ (1)} + \tfrac{3}{4}O_2 \text{ (g)} \rightarrow Au(OH)_3 \text{ (S)} \quad \Delta G° = +65,700$$

In this reaction the free energy is positive and it indicates that the reaction has no intensity to go at all and gold, correspondingly, does not corrode in aqueous media. Media to form $Au(OH)_3$.

Note: The tendency to corrode does not measure the rate of reaction.

Pilling-Bedworth Ratio

Pilling-Bedworth ratio is a parameter applied to estimate the extent of oxidation that happened in a system. It can be defined as Md/nmD, where D is density and Mare molecular weight of the corrosion product scale that forms on the metal surface during oxidation; d and m are the density and atomic weight respectively of the metal and n is a number of metal atoms in a molecular formula of scale, e.g. for Al_2O_3, n = 2. Pilling and Bedworth ratio judge the volume of the corrosion product whether it was greater or less than the volume of the metal from which the corrosion is formed.

If Md/nm D < 1, this tells that volume of corrosion product that formed is less than the volume of metal from which the product is formed. Md/nm D > 1, if the volume is greater than 1, the corrosion product scale is greater than the volume of metal from which the scale it formed, so that scale is in protective, compression of the underlying metal. Pilling-Bedworth ratio must be Md/nm D >>1, the scale that forms may buckle and detach from the surface because of the higher stresses that develop. In the case of aluminium, the Pilling-Bedworth ratio is 1:3, so it corrodes slowly, as it forms a protective oxide, and whereas magnesium, which tends to form non-protective oxides, the ratio is 0:8.

CORROSION MONITORING AND TECHNIQUES USED IN OBSERVATION

Many definitions are coined to describe the corrosion monitoring since, the industrial corrosion techniques are used and applied to overcome the problem of corrosion. Some of the definitions of corrosion monitoring are as follows:

- "Techniques which use to observe and monitor the progress of corrosion"
- "The systemic measurement of the corrosion or degradation of an item of equipment, with the objective of assisting the understanding of the corrosion process and obtaining information for use in controlling corrosion and its consequences."

The knowledge of assessment of the degradation of a material caused by chemical, environment, biological and electrochemical reaction, it provides the mechanisms.

The objectives on which the corrosion monitoring studies are based as follows:

- To detect the corrosion in the beginning stage and action can be taken to reduce or stop it in operating equipment
- To control, monitor, assess and report the effectiveness of corrosion risk and mitigation processes such as inhibitor addition on working machinery.

Techniques and Processes Used in Corrosion Monitoring the Corrosion

Choice of techniques depends on the corrosion type, as its investigation includes different methods that need to be followed while monitoring the corrosion. To see that the method used to monitor the corrosion is appropriate or not, compatibility with any existing techniques that are used in inspection and monitoring. When inspection is done, it must be defined for what purpose and monitoring it is used like invasive (penetrating into equipment) or non-invasive (when measurement made without any penetration), continuous (with data available with continuously probes) and periodic (sensors exposed to the process but which need to extracted for analysis such as corrosion coupons). Some techniques which are used in monitoring are:

- Coupons
- Electrical resistance (ER)
- Electrochemical techniques:
  - Potential measurement
  - Potentiodynamic/cyclic polarization
  - Linear polarization resistance (LPR)
  - Galvanic current
  - Electrochemical impedance spectroscopy (EIS)
  - Electrochemical noise (EN)
- Field signature method (FSM)
- Thin layer activation
- Chemical analysis
- Hydrogen
- Test heat exchangers and spool pieces
- Monitoring of bacteria
- Thickness inspection and measurement of crack detection
- Sentinel holes
- Visual inspection.

METHODS OF PREVENTION AND CONTROLLING OF CORROSION

In prevention and controlling the corrosion, there are many factors and steps need to be followed like plant and process design, construction stage checks, planned maintenance, corrosion monitoring, and remedial action and diagnostic work. All these factors need to consider for the betterment and smooth functioning of the working plant, as these steps will also control the harmful effects of the degradation that take place by corrosion. By these measures, the cost and maintenance can be reduced.

Plant and Process Design

It involves the affecting of the materials of construction, process conditions, equipment design, and recommended operating practices to avoid the risk of corrosion. While designing a pilot plant, an internal project team may design the plant, with all the required procedures and precautions need to be taken or it can be forwarded by the contractors and its design will be reviewed by the expert before construction. Therefore corrosion engineer must be involved from the inception of the project. A simple block design of phase of corrosion control Fig. 11.3.

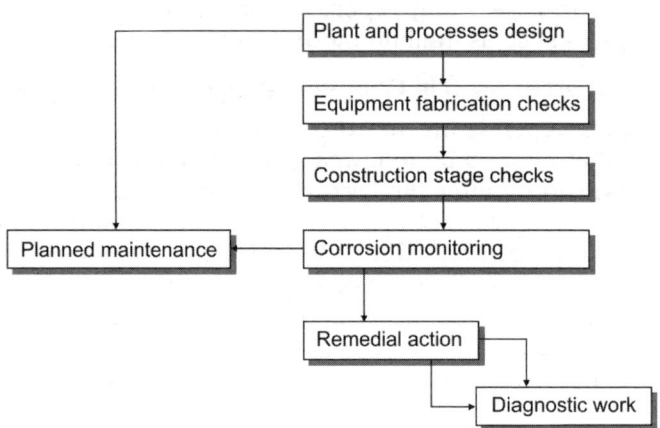

Fig. 11.3: Phase of corrosion control

Further use of some other technologically advanced materials can also prohibit or delay the corrosion like using Corrosion-Resistant Alloy (CRA) with several other combinations of the metal to special CRAs, e.g. nickel-chromium-molybdenum (Ni-Cr-Mo) alloys, molybdenum, in combination with chromium, increase the resistance to pitting and crevice corrosion. And also stabilises the passive film in the presence of chlorides.

A piping design consideration is also very important as they come with many critical and predicted fouls, the major three problems recorded are dead legs, high velocities and water traps. The place at low sections of the piping system where water stagnates and accumulates causing corrosion is known as the water traps which are the first area to be inspected.

Pitting corrosion is the most frequently occurring corrosion mechanisms at water traps can be possible to minimise low sections by any of methods, such as slanting the pipe or by installing drain valves at the low points that are periodically drained. It may occur in environments where stagnant particles are deposited on a metal surface, as initiated, the pits grow until they penetrate through the metal wall, causing a leak which is especially dangerous in pressurised systems because a leak may release aggressive or flammable chemicals under high pressure. The regions of the piping system where the fluid is stagnant are called dead legs. It can be minimised in the piping by providing drains so that stagnant deposits can be flushed, by designing pipes with elbows rather than turning the complete pipelining or by placing valves to have the shortest dead legs, by placing branch lines off from the top rather than from the side.

Velocity effects causes cavitation and erosion-corrosion. Cavitation corrosion is caused when vapour bubbles are collapse and formed in a fluid medium due to changes in pressure. It may cause significant wall loss at the site where the bubbles impact on the metal. Erosion-corrosion is caused when the protective scale of a metal is removed due to high-velocity flow or turbulence. Erosion-corrosion may occur at elbows, tees and internal protrusions, such as valves and weld beads. However, process changes over time and may change the fluid volume transported through the piping therefore, the piping which carries the fluid piping should be designed with large diameters to transport the required material.

Construction Stage Checks

The construction area needs to check with a valid inspection system to make sure that fabricators are functioning according to the design pattern and codes. The operating system working with that system is having extensive value in inspection required. The standard operating procedure at construction stage should be checked for each material supplied. The repair and treatment carried out for those wrong and damaged materials. The mistake happens due to following reasons:

1. Assembled products were mixed and a mixup happened from supplier side due to the confusion as many materials have same design and appearances (identity system).
2. Valves, welding electrodes and piping usually get mixed up due to the poor identification marking and moreover they are always supplied in large units (poor identification system).

Any pre-treatment to the equipment should be specified by a standard operating procedure like descaling must be carried out before the use. All this should be mentioned to the fabricator because sometimes unusually some accident can take place which results in materials lost or other safety issues. The details that are mentioned make a working smooth and the minimum trouble during the early operational period of a new plant.

Planned Maintenance

A planned and proper time-table of the maintenance and regular replacement or services of the plant machinery and equipment need for the better functioning and to avoid any failure be the mean of corrosion, etc. This is also an important adjunct to design and constitutes the 3rd phase of control. The design should be emphasised on controlling and minimising the occurrence of corrosion, but if these precautions are failed to achieve then additional capital need to invest for prevention of the corrosion. Planned maintenance consists of scheduled shutdown periods in order to inspect all equipment and refurnish or replace equipment that has failed due to corrosion or other failure mechanisms. The shutdown periods are generally scheduled well in advance. The shutdowns are short in duration since inspection costs and production losses are the determining cost factors for the economic value of the scheduled shutdown. In the pharmaceutical industry, process tanks, pipes, and valves are routinely electropolished to reduce the adhesion of a product and to decrease the risk of bacterial growth in crevices. The packaging of pharmaceutical products is also important in order to minimise damage due to corrosion by split products; therefore, desiccant bags filled with highly active drying materials are often used as a means of protection. In addition, the atmosphere inside the packaging can be maintained at a level of relatively low humidity so that corrosion can be avoided.

Remedial Action and Diagnostic Work

Corrosion monitoring sometimes also involves the fifth phase of control which is known as a remedial action and diagnostic work to be effective. In some cases of corrosion the remedial measure is known and can be easily deduced. However, in others the diagnostic work has to precede a decision on a remedial action. Some of the remedial measures that are taken as follows—change equipment design, install cathodic protection system, install anodic protection system, improve feedstock purity, alter process variables, change materials and institute inhibitor additions.

BASICS OF MATERIAL HANDLING SYSTEMS

Material handling system is one of the basic components of any manufacturing unit/ system. It can be defined as the procedure or an activity which involves the movement, storage, protecting, control of materials, disposal, distribution and consumption in a defined system. In a material handling, series technical activities are used like manual, semi-automated and automated instruments. One of the definitions adopted way back by the American Materials Handling Society is: Materials handling is the art and science involving the moving, packaging and storing of substances in any form. The definition can further understood with their role in the industries like delivering the right amount of material at the right place within the right time in the right position followed by right sequence in a right cost. Material handling done in a system or sequence will lead to help in resource allocation, production planning, flow and process management, forecasting, inventory management and control, support and service with satisfied customer delivery.

Material handling further involves these machinery or equipment that are responsible for the material movements. These systems used in the type of industries are chemical, beverages, pharmaceuticals, e-commerce, food, hardwares, hospital, manufacturing (material processing), paper mill, plastics, retails, warehousing and distribution. They are categories as:
- Automatic guided vehicles
- Automated storage
- Automated retrieval systems
- Data collection and identification through used of automatic system
- Controls of caster and wheels, conveyer belt
- Dock equipment
- Ergonomics
- Industrial robots; full automated and self-driven (lift trucks, monorail and work stations cranes, overhead cranes)
- Cohesive material handling units
- Inventory tally system (audit system)
- Packaging (protective guarding system)
- Storage (racks, shelves, air tight close box, humidity free chambers)
- Software (multitasking)
- Sortation (allocation of items according to their appropriate place therefore avoid mixing of materials).

In order to perform the activities of materials handling the basic goal is to minimize the production costs. This general objective can be further subdivided into specific objectives as follows:
- To reduce the costs by decreasing inventories, minimizing the distance to be handled and increasing productivity
- To increase the production capacity by smoothing the work flow
- To minimize the waste during handling
- To improve distribution through better location of facilities and improved routing

- To increase the equipment and space utilization
- To improve the working conditions
- To improve the customer service.

Four Major Types of Materials Handling Methods

1. **Movement:** It involves the actual transportation or transfer of material from one point to the next.
2. **Quantity:** Dictates the type and nature of the material handling equipment and also cost per unit for the conveyance of the goods.
3. **Time:** How quickly, the material can move through the facility space-concerned with the required space for the storage of the material handling equipment and their movement, as well as the queuing or staging space for the material itself.
4. **Control:** Racking of the material, positive identification, and inventory management. A major competitive advantage due to its impact on quality, cost, productivity, inventory, and response time; in total a revenue enhancer not a cost contributor.

For a material handling system the design must be in a way that all the systems like manual and automated systems should work in unified system with a defined protocol. There are many principle of material handling which are considered before initiating any handling and transfer of the material this ensure the safety and improves customer satisfaction and services, while reducing the faults like longer time delivery, errors in delivery, lowering the cost of handling and utilising, transport and distribution. The principles can be categories as:

- **Orientation principle:** It encourages study of all available system relationships before moving towards preliminary planning. The study includes looking at existing methods, problems, etc.
- **Planning principle:** It establishes a plan which includes basic requirements, desirable alternates and planning for contingency
- **Systems principle:** It integrates handling and storage activities, which is cost effective into integrated system design
- **Unit load principle:** Handle product in a unit load as large as possible
- **Space utilization principle:** Encourage effective utilization of all the space available
- **Standardization principle:** It encourages standardization of handling methods and equipment
- **Ergonomic principle:** It recognizes human capabilities and limitation by design effective handling equipment
- **Energy principle:** It considers consumption of energy during material handling
- **Ecology principle:** It encourages minimum impact upon the environment during material handling
- **Mechanization principle:** It encourages mechanization of handling process wherever possible as to encourage efficiency
- **Flexibility principle:** Encourages of methods and equipment which are possible to utilize in all types of condition
- **Simplification principle:** Encourage simplification of methods and process by removing unnecessary movements
- **Gravity principle:** Encourages usage of gravity principle in movement of goods

- **Safety principle:** Encourages provision for safe handling equipment according to safety rules and regulation
- **Computerization principle:** Encourages computerization of material handling and storage systems
- **System flow principle:** Encourages integration of data flow with physical material flow
- **Layout principle:** Encourages preparation of operational sequence of all systems available
- **Cost principle:** Encourages cost benefit analysis of all solutions available
- **Maintenance principle:** Encourages preparation of plan for preventive maintenance and scheduled repairs
- **Obsolescence principle:** Encourage preparation of equipment policy as to enjoy appropriate economic advantage.

CHARACTERISTICS AND CLASSIFICATION OF MATERIALS

Method to be adopted and choice of equipment for a materials handling system primarily depends on the type of material/s to be handled. It is therefore, very important to know about different types of materials and their characteristics which are related to methods and equipment used for their handling. As innumerable different materials are used and need to be handled in industries, they are classified based on specific characteristics relevant to their handling. Basic classification of material is made on the basis of **forms**, which are **(i) Gases, (ii) Liquids, (iii) Semi Liquids and (iv) Solids**. Following characteristics of gases, liquids and semiliquids are relevant to their handling. For gases it is primarily pressure, high (25 psi and more) or low (<25 psi). Chemical properties are also important. For liquids the relevant characteristics are density, viscosity, freezing and boiling point, corrosiveness, temperature, inflammability, etc. Examples of common industrial liquids are: water, mineral oils, acids, alkalis, chemicals, etc. Examples of common semi-liquids are: slurry, sewage, sludge, mud, pulp, paste, etc. Gases are generally handled in tight and where required, pressure resisting containers. However, most common method of handling of large volume of gas is through pipes by the help of compressor, blower, etc. This process is known as pneumatic conveying. Liquids and semi-liquids can be handled in tight or open containers which may be fitted with facilities like insulation, heating, cooling, agitating, etc. as may be required by the character of the liquid. Large quantity of stable liquids/semiliquids are generally conveyed through pipes using suitable pumps, which is commonly known as hydraulic conveying. Solids form the majority of materials which are handled in industrial situation. Solids are classified into two main groups: Unit load and Bulk load (materials).

Unit loads are formed solids of various sizes, shapes and weights. Some of these are counted by number of pieces like machine parts, molding boxes and fabricated items. Tared goods like containers, bags, packaged items, etc. and materials which are handled en-masses like forest products (logs), structurals, pig iron, etc. are other examples of unit loads. The specific characteristics of unit loads are their over all dimensions, shape, piece-weight, temperature, inflammability, strength/fragility, etc. Hoisting equipment and trucks are generally used for handling unit loads. Certain types of conveyors are also used particularly for cartons/packaged items and metallic long-products like angles, rods, etc. Unit loads have been classified by Bureau of Indian Standards' (BIS) specification number IS 8005:1976(2).

The classifications are based on:

- **Shape of unit loads**—(*i*) basic geometric forms like rectangular, cylindrical, pyramidal/conical and spherical; (*ii*) typical or usual forms like pallets, plate, containers, bales and sacks; (*iii*) irregular forms like objects with flat base dimension smaller than overall size, loads on rollers/wheels and uneven shapes
- **Position of CG (stability) of load**
- **Mass of unit load** in 10 steps from 0–2.5 kg to more than 5000 kg
- **Volume per unit** in 10 steps from 0–10 cm^3 to more than 10 m^3
- **Type of material** in contact with conveying system like metal, wood, paper/ cardboard, textile, rubber/plastics, glass and other materials
- **Geometrical shape** (flat, concave, convex, irregular/uneven, ribbed, etc.) and **physical properties** (smooth, slippery, rough, hard, elastic, etc.) **of base surface of unit load**
- **Specific physical and chemical properties** of unit loads like abrasive, corrosive, dust emitting, damp, greasy/oily, hot, cold, fragile, having sharp edges, inflammable, explosive, hygroscopic, sticky, toxic, obnoxious, radioactive, etc.
- **Loads sensitive** to pressure, shock, vibration, turning/tilting, acceleration/ deceleration, cold, heat, light, radiation, damp, etc.

Bulk materials are those which are powdery, granular or lumpy in nature and are stored in heaps. Example of bulk materials are minerals (ores, coals, etc.), earthy materials (gravel, sand, clay, etc.) processed materials (cement, salt, chemicals, etc.), agricultural products (grain, sugar, flour, etc.) and similar other materials.

Major characteristics of bulk materials, so far as their handling is concerned, are: lump-size, bulk weight, specific weight, moisture content, flowability (mobility of its particles), angles of repose, abrasiveness, temperature, proneness to explosion, stickiness, fuming or dusty, corrosivity, hygroscopic, etc. Lump size of a material is determined by the distribution of particle sizes. If the largest to smallest size ratio of the particles of a lumpy material is above 2.5, they are considered to be unsized.

The average lump size of sized bulk material
$$= 1/2 \text{ (maximum particle size + minimum particle size)}$$
$$= 1/2 \text{ (}a\text{ max} + a\text{ min)}$$

Bulk weight or bulk density of a lumpy material is the weight of the material per unit volume in bulk. Because of empty spaces within the particles in bulk materials, bulk density is always less than density of a particle of the same material. Generally bulk load can be packed by static or dynamic loading. The ratio of the bulk density of a packed material to its bulk density before packing is known as the **packing coefficient** whose value varies for different bulk materials and their lump size, from 1.05 to 1.52. Bulk density is generally expressed in kg/m^3.

Mobility or **flowability** of a bulk material is generally determined by its **angle of repose**. When a bulk materialis freely spilled over a horizontal plane, it assumes a conical heap. The angle ϕ of the cone with the horizontal plane is called the angle of repose. Less is ϕ, higher is the flowability of the bulk material. If the heap is shaken, the heap becomes flatter and the corresponding angle of repose under dynamic condition is referred to as dynamic angle of repose ϕ dyne, where ϕ dyne is generally considered to be equal to 0.7ϕ. Classification and codification of bulk materials based on lump size, flowability, abrasiveness, bulk density and various other characteristics have been specified by the BIS specification number IS:8730:1997(3).

The alphanumeric codification system as per this specification is shown below:

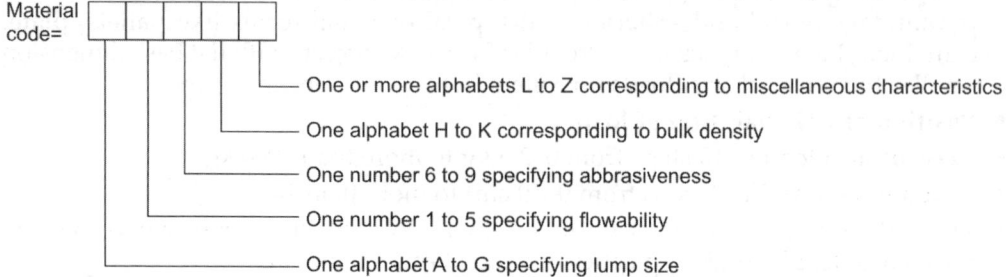

In this material code, if any of the above characteristics is not known, corresponding number or alphabet is dropped from the material code.

Advantages of Materials Handling

- Savings in storage and operating space
- Better stock control
- Improved working conditions
- Improved quality
- Lower risk of accidents
- Reduced processing time
- Lower production costs
- Less waste of time and materials.

Disadvantages of Material Handling

- Additional capital cost involved in any materials handling system
- Once a materials handling system get implemented, flexibility for further changes gets greatly reduced
- With an integrated materials handling system installed, failure/stoppage in any portion of it leads to increased down time of the production system
- Materials handling system needs maintenance, hence any addition to materials handling means additional maintenance facilities and costs.

VERY SHORT QUESTIONS

1. Explain the use of glass lined equipment in the pharmaceutical plant.
2. Explain the importance of stainless steel in pharmaceutical plant.
3. Name five important classes of plastics and its applications.
4. How does addition of amines protect against corrosion of iron?
5. Explain the role of oxygen and pH on corrosion.
6. Define the following:
   a. Pitting corrosion
   b. Galvanic corrosion
   c. Chemical corrosion
   d. Corrosion fatigue

SHORT QUESTIONS

1. Mention all the characteristics of materials.

2. List important type of glass containers. Mention an example of formulation that is stored in each type of container.

3. Describe steel and rubber used as a material of construction.

4. Write a note on alloys used in pharmacy practice.

5. What is corrosion? Mention factors affecting rate of corrosion.

6. Differentiate between:
   a. Ferrous and non-ferrous metals
   b. Inorganic and organic non-metals

LONG QUESTIONS

1. Enlist the factors affecting during materials selection for pharmaceutical plant construction.

2. Write the theories of corrosion in detail.

3. Enumerate the types of corrosion and there prevention methods used in pharmaceutical plant.

4. Explain the types and principles of material handling systems.

5. What is material? State its characteristics and importance in pharmaceutical plant.

MULTIPLE CHOICE QUESTIONS

1. In equipment design, the following factor/s is/are considered:
   a. Materials of selection
   b. Safety factors
   c. Both A and B
   d. None

2. Corrosion of metals involves
   a. Physical reactions
   b. Chemical reactions
   c. Both
   d. None

3. Which of the following factors play vital role in corrosion process?
   a. Temperature
   b. Solute concentration
   c. Both
   d. None

4. Which of the following equation is related to corrosion rate?
   a. Nernst equation
   b. Faraday's equation
   c. Either
   d. Neither

5. Select the incorrect statement from the following option:
   a. Replacement of corroded equipment is time-consuming
   b. Corrosion causes contamination of product
   c. Corrosion increases the electrical conductivity of metals
   d. Corrosion causes leakage of toxic liquid or gases

6. **Leakage of inflammable gas from corroded pipe can cause:**
   a. Acidity
   b. Alkalinity
   c. Turbidity
   d. Fire hazards

7. **The process of deterioration of a metal due to unwanted chemical or electrochemical interaction of metal with its environment is called:**
   a. Electrolysis
   b. Electrodialysis
   c. Corrosion
   d. Deposition

8. **Which of the following is an example of corrosion?**
   a. Rusting of iron
   b. Tarnishing of silver
   c. Liquefaction of ammonia
   d. Rusting of iron and tarnishing of silver

9. **Process of corrosion enhanced by:**
   a. AIR and moisture
   b. Electrolytes in water
   c. Metallic impurities
   d. All of above

10. **Stainless steel contains:**
    a. 10% vanadium, 8% chromium
    b. 18% chromium, 8% nickel
    c. 18% tungsten, 8% nickel
    d. 18% tungsten, 8% chromium

11. **Shock resistance of steel is increased by adding:**
    a. Nickel
    b. Sulphur, lead and phosphorus
    c. Nickel and chromium
    d. None

12. **Material handling consists of movement of material from:**
    a. One machine to another
    b. One shop to another shop
    c. Stores to shop
    d. All of the above

13. **Economy in material handling can be achieved by:**
    a. Employing gravity feed movements
    b. Minimizing distance of travel
    c. By carrying material to destination without using manual labour
    d. All of the above

14. **Principle of 'Unit load' states that:**
    a. Materials should be moved in lots
    b. One unit should be moved at a time
    c. Both 'a' and 'b'
    d. None of the above

15. **What type of glass is used for the preparation of distill water stills?**
    a. Jena glass
    b. Soft glass
    c. Hard glass
    d. Quartz glass

16. **Protection against IR can be achieved using one of the following containers**
    a. Amber coloured
    b. Transparent
    c. Yellow coloured
    d. Green coloured

17. **Which one of the following can retard the corrosion of metals:**
    a. Carbon   b. Chromium
    c. Zinc   d. Iron

18. **Type of corrosion of metals related to flow is:**
    a. Erosion   b. Biological corrosion
    c. Crevice corrosion   d. Intergranular corrosion

19. **Material handling method involves:**
    a. Time   b. Movement
    c. Both a and b   d. None

20. **Rubber contains one of the following chemical units:**
    a. Amino acid   b. Sugar
    c. Isoprene   d. Glycosidal

Index